LIFE AFTER COVID-19

LIFE AFTER COVID-19

LESSONS FROM PAST PANDEMICS

BOB GORDON

BANOVALLUM
BOOKS

Published in Great Britain in 2020
by Banovallum Books
an imprint of Mortons Books Ltd.
Media Centre
Morton Way
Horncastle LN9 6JR
www.mortonsbooks.co.uk

ISBN 978 1 911658 77 1

The right of Bob Gordon to be identified as the author of this work
has been asserted in accordance with the Copyright, Designs and
Patents Act 1988.

Typeset by BookEmpress Ltd., London
Printed and bound by Gutenberg Press, Malta

Acknowledgements

Writing during a pandemic lockdown the list is short. Elena Cremonese at the Halifax Municipal Archives went above and beyond. Daryl Grennan handled all the computer problems a techno-peasant couldn't. The cast and crew at Mortons were all supportive and provided excellent editorial guidance. As ever, Frank and Glenys' friendship was invaluable.

CONTENTS

Introduction

"History is a vast early warning system."
Norman Cousins, American journalist, author and editor
(June 24, 1915-November 30, 1990)

A T A FEW minutes after 10am on Tuesday, November 1, 2005, President George W. Bush, one year into his second term, strode to the podium at the William Natcher Center at the Bethesda, Maryland headquarters of the National Institutes of Health (NIH). Among those in the audience was Dr Anthony Fauci, who was then and remains at the time of writing the director of the National Institute of Allergy and Infectious Diseases.

After the requisite formalities, the president got straight to the point: "At this moment, the men and women of the NIH are working to protect the American people from another danger – the risk of avian and pandemic influenza... I'm here to discuss our strategy to prevent and protect the American people from a possible outbreak." Bush was speaking in the shadow of SARS (Severe Acute Respiratory Syndrome – of which there had been outbreaks in 2002 and 2004, both originating in China).

"A pandemic is a lot like a forest fire. If caught early it might be extinguished with limited damage. If allowed to smolder, undetected, it can grow to an inferno that can spread quickly beyond our ability to control it. To respond to a pandemic, we need medical personnel and adequate supplies of equipment. In a pandemic, everything from syringes to hospital beds, respirators masks and protective equipment would be in short supply.

"If a pandemic strikes, our country must have a surge capacity in place that will allow us to bring a new vaccine on line quickly and manufacture enough to immunise every American against the pandemic strain."

The catastrophic pandemic he was warning his audience about, SARS-CoV-2 (Severe Acute Respiratory Syndrome Coronavirus 2 – the virus that causes the COVID-19 disease), finally struck in 2020. Its existence was first noted on December 31, 2019, when Wuhan Municipal Health Commission, China, reported a cluster of pneumonia cases in Wuhan, Hubei Province. On New Year's Day the Wuhan wet market, a market selling live animals, both wild and domestic, was closed as a suspected source of the outbreak.

The World Health Organization (WHO), based in Geneva, Switzerland, set up an incident management support team the following day and reported the Wuhan outbreak via social media on January 4, 2020, stating that there had been no deaths. The first recorded case outside China was identified in Thailand on January 13 and on January 30 the WHO declared a Public Health Emergency of International Concern. A situation report issued on the same day stated that 7818 cases had been confirmed worldwide.

On January 31, US President Donald Trump banned most travel from China to the United States. He delayed the arrival of the virus on US shores, but there was no chance that he could prevent it. It is doubtful that Trump and his team fully understood the potential threat since his administration undertook only minimal preparations.

The president's own words speak for themselves. Throughout the first half of March he repeatedly expressed shock and amazement at the rapid spread of the virus. On March 6 he described it as "an unforeseen problem. What a problem. Came out of nowhere." The following week, on March 11, the same day that the WHO categorised COVID-19 a pandemic, he told the nation's bankers: "We're having to fix a problem that, four weeks ago, nobody ever thought it would be a problem. Nobody."

At an official press briefing of the Coronavirus Task Force on March 14 he asserted, again, "It's something that nobody expected." The president was mistaken. He would have been closer to the truth if he had said instead, 'It's something that nobody, in my administration, expected.'

Indeed, a devastating pandemic was foreseen by many people, who had been roundly dismissed by the Trump administration and, to be fair, by most governments in Europe and North America. Canada had received a direct warning in 2003 when Toronto was one of only a handful of cities to face an outbreak of SARS. Nonetheless, 17 years later the Canadian government was caught flat-footed by COVID-19.

Lack of preparedness despite the wild ringing of alarm bells is nothing new, however. Throughout the four centuries following the introduction of bubonic plague to Europe in 1347, it had periodically reappeared and ravaged the continent. Yet it continued to catch authorities off guard – it was as though every time the disease died down, everyone was only too happy to simply forget about it.

In his account of the Great Plague of London in 1665, A Journal of the Plague Year, published in 1722, novelist Daniel Defoe wrote, "Surely never city, at least, of this bulk and magnitude, was taken in a condition so perfectly unprepar'd for such a dreadful visitation, whether I am to speak of the civil preparations, or religious; they were indeed, as if they had had no warning, no expectation, no apprehensions, and consequently the least provision imaginable, was made for it in a publick way." Half a century after the fact he was still warning of a plague he felt no one else was preparing for.

Unfortunately, there is nothing sexy about procuring and storing thousands of ventilators and millions of N95/P3 masks for an unknown threat that might never materialise. Pandemics make for great movies, but they are not great politics. When 'not in my lifetime' is a widely held belief and political lives are measured in months not decades, politicians are disinclined to invest in a once-in-a-century cataclysm.

Three years before the 2020 coronavirus pandemic Jeremy Konyndyk, former director of USAID's Office of US Foreign Disaster Assistance, gave a prescient warning, "A major new global health crisis is a question of when, not if… At some point a highly fatal, highly contagious virus will emerge – like the 1918 'Spanish flu' pandemic, which infected one third of the world's population and killed between 50 and 100 million people." Given the qua-drupling of the global population in the last century that would amount to between 200 and 400 million dead, today. Pessimistically, Konyndyk also pre-dicted that this new crisis would be sorely mishandled by the Trump admin-istration when it happened.

Even more recently, agencies within the United States government were broadcasting concerns about the increasing likelihood of a new pandemic. In February 2018, the Worldwide Threat Assessment of the US Intelligence Community stated, there is the "potential for a severe global health emer-gency… with pathogens such as H5N1 and H7N9 influenza and Middle East Respiratory Syndrome Coronavirus having pandemic potential if they were to acquire efficient human-to-human transmissibility." A year later the warning was repeated, "the United States and the world will remain vulner-able to the next flu pandemic or large-scale outbreak of a contagious dis-ease…" Scientists, academics, bureaucrats and political allies and critics were all sounding the alarm about a pandemic, most about a viral pandemic, some as specific as a coronavirus pandemic.

This is hardly surprising. Historians have been writing about periodic pandemics and their profound consequences for millennia. The historian Thucydides (460/455 to 399/398 BCE) documented an Athenian plague that killed Pericles, a leading statesmen, in 429 BCE. The Greek physician Galen, living in Rome, chronicled the Antoinine plague in the last half of the second century CE. Englishman Samuel Pepys (pronounced Peeps) dia-ried and Dafoe documented the Great Plague of London in the 1660s and Boccaccio's Decameron of 1353 opens with excruciating descriptions of the physical agonies of victims of the Black Death. The first cholera pandemic even makes an appearance in the Narrative of the Life of Frederick Douglass, an American Slave, published in 1845. The COVID-19 pandemic is caused by a virus new to the human population but pandemics of varying frequency and ferocity have blighted the historical record from the very beginning.

In strictly medical terms, these past pandemics have little to offer that may be of use today. The 2020 outbreak resulted from a virus while cholera is a bacterial illness, as is bubonic plague. Mode of transmission has been dissimilar too. Fleas carried bubonic plague from rats to humans while chol-era was transmitted through water contaminated by human waste (the pesky microbe, hell bent on increasing its likelihood of surviving and reproducing, induces in its victims endless diarrhea so severe it can cause death by dehydration, but greatly increasing its virulence). The novel coronavirus is, like influenza, a virus rather than a bacteria.

And medical technology and techniques have advanced by leaps and bounds in the century since the Spanish flu. It is almost absurd to compare the practices, as involved as they were ineffective, used to treat or prevent the horrible hard lymph nodes and black buboes of the plague with today's medical procedures. But for all its advances, today's medical science is, at the time of writing, almost as impotent when it comes to treating COVID-19.

The present day generation faces a frightening situation that would have been intimately familiar to our medieval forebears. Little is known for certain about the disease – the precise mode of transmission, the length of time infectiousness can endure, the human body's reaction to it. It is all unknown territory and everyone everywhere was forced to adopt practices in 2020 which, again, would not have seemed out of place to any of our ancestors who had any familiarity with an outbreak of disease: social distancing, travel bans – even stockpiling.

One other factor would also be familiar. The essential, elemental similarity of all pandemics is a rapidly escalating fatality rate. Regardless of their etiology, vectors and other differences all pandemics cause death and depopulation, resulting in social dislocation and economic disruption. For this reason they can offer important insights into the aftermath of medical disasters and, perhaps, the future – the world after the COVID-19 pandemic.

To that end, considering historic pandemics can prove fruitful. The Black Death, a misnomer, swept mid-14th century Europe killing roughly half of the population. It deservedly lays claim to being the grand-daddy of all pandemics. Subsequently, bubonic plague remained endemic in Europe with periodic outbreaks and epidemics. In 1665-66 the Great Plague of London killed approximately one-quarter of the city's population of 460,000.

After breaking out of India in 1817, in the half century after 1832, cholera repeatedly visited western Europe and North America particularly ravaging immigrants in transit and on their arrival. Cholera's emergence occurred at a revolutionary time in medical science and it was largely 'defeated' (again, in terms of Europe and North America) over the 19th century. One hundred years ago the Spanish Flu pandemic, another misnomer, claimed between 50m and 100m lives globally. After four years of savage warfare with casualties in numbers never seen before, a pandemic added to the butcher's bill. In each case the etiology and course of the disease, its treatment, its virulence and its morbidity will be outlined. However, the emphasis will not be on the medical aspect of pandemics, but rather, their aftershocks.

Ultimately, the current pandemic will be considered. Again, the medical aspects of the current crisis will be outlined. However, the focus is on the future. What kind of a world will emerge after this pandemic? And, more specifically, what can past pandemics tell us about the aftermath of this one? Two issues will be studiously avoided: the question of whether the world's governments were sufficiently prepared is redundant. Of course they were not; the hundreds of thousands of dead provide mute testimony to that. Why, and who was responsible for that situation, along with grading the performance of individual politicians, professionals and bureaucrats is outside the scope of this book.

Suffice to say that pandemic planners – politicians, bureaucrats and scientists – face a deadly Catch-22. Mike Leavitt, a name long forgotten by most was, once, a favourite target of late night comics. Why? During the Avian Flu epidemic, as George W. Bush's Secretary of Health in 2006 he recommended US citizens stock up on non-perishable food items in preparation for an epidemic and lockdown. On the Tonight Show, Jay Leno quipped: "Secretary of Health and Human Services Michael Leavitt recommended that Americans store canned tuna and powdered milk under their beds for when bird flu hits. What? … Powdered milk and tuna? How many would rather have the bird flu?" Ridiculed for advocating preparedness he recently told the website Politico, "In advance of a pandemic, anything you say sounds alarmist. After a pandemic starts, everything you've done is inadequate."

A glossary is included to acquaint the reader with various medical and epidemiological terms. However, certain introductory terms demand immediate definition. 'Plague' has multiple uses and meanings currently. One can refer to an ongoing plague of locusts in eastern Africa. As a verb, one can be plagued by Internet trolls. In these senses, plague has become a generic term for something bothersome that is numerous or repetitive. However, in a medical sense plague has a very precise meaning, referring to a specific disease. According to Oxford, plague is, "a contagious bacterial disease characterized by fever and delirium, typically with the formation of buboes (bubonic plague) and sometimes infection of the lungs (pneumonic plague)." Plague, specifically, bubonic plague is a particular disease, one that reached epidemic proportions during the period (1347-53) that we commonly, and incorrectly call, the 'Black Death' and again, in London, three centuries later. However, neither cholera, a distinct bacterial infection, nor COVID19, a viral infection, can be properly referred to as plague.

It is also essential to understand the differences between the terms endemic, epidemic and pandemic. According to the Centre for Disease Control (CDC) in Atlanta, endemic refers to the baseline or 'normal' frequency of a given disease within a given population or geographical region. For example, between 2000 and 2017 Canada, with a population of 30m to 35m, averaged approximately 20,000 cases of flu annually and 18 flu deaths per season, with a high of 21 and a low of 15. Ideally, of course, there would be no flu deaths but the endemic level of a disease is not the ideal – it is the reality.

An epidemic is defined as a sudden and rapid spike above the endemic level in the incidence of a disease in a given area. If Canada had seen 200,000 cases and hundreds of deaths in a single year during the aforementioned time period, that year would have constituted an epidemic, a significant, rapid increase from endemic levels. The virulence and mortality rate of an illness are not factors in defining it as an epidemic, only rapidly increasing frequency, a sudden departure from endemic levels, define an epidemic. In January 2020, one could describe COVID-19 as an epidemic of limited geographic scope restricted to China or, even more specifically, Hubei province or the city of Wuhan.

A pandemic is an epidemic that has spread rapidly to multiple countries and continents. When WHO Director-General Tedros Adhanom Ghebreyesus, an Ethiopian microbiologist and internationally recognized malaria researcher, declared COVID-19 a pandemic on March 11, 2020, he said: "In the past two weeks, the number of cases of COVID-19 outside China has increased 13-fold, and the number of affected countries has tripled. There are now more than 118,000 cases in 114 countries, and 4291 people have lost their lives... We have therefore made the assessment that

COVID-19 can be characterised as a pandemic." The WHO was criticized for making this call too late. However, as Ghebreyesus added, "Describing the situation as a pandemic does not change WHO's assessment of the threat posed by this virus. It doesn't change what WHO is doing, and it doesn't change what countries should do." COVID-19 was an epidemic that grew into a pandemic.

It is equally important to differentiate between the novel coronavirus and COVID-19. The former is the virus that causes the illness known as COVID-19. It is analogous to the term HIV/AIDS. HIV (Human Immunodeficiency Virus) is the virus that causes AIDS (Acquired Immune Deficiency Syndrome) and in a similar fashion, the bacterium called Vibrio cholerae causes cholera.

These microbes bear the human species no ill will; in every pandemic the microbe is just doing its thing: trying to survive long enough to reproduce. From homo sapiens to the Yersinia pestis coccobacillus bacterium, that biological imperative drives every living creature. Microbes, while they are making us ill, even killing us, are simply fulfilling their biological function.

To this end, successful microbes evolve an entire arsenal. Pride of place belongs to the rabies virus. Transferred via an animal's saliva, it actually changes their behaviour, inducing a biting frenzy to facilitate transmission. A virus that promptly overwhelms and kills its host, kills itself. Many viruses, notably HIV, have evolved to keep their hosts alive much longer. This prolongs the virus's life and increases its opportunity to procreate and infect new hosts.

As noted earlier, cholera bacteria is shed in profusion by a sufferer's diarrhea, an ideal vector to the next host via their drinking water. COVID-19 is spread by airborne droplets that are projected with autonomic force when we cough, sneeze and laugh. Consider American historian Jared Diamond's charming description of a sexually transmitted disease: "From our perspective, the open genital sores caused by venereal diseases like syphilis are a vile indignity. From the microbe's point of view, however, they are just a useful device to enlist a host's help in inoculating microbes into a body cavity of a new host." From the virus's point of view, how it affects a human body, whether the human host lives or dies, is meaningless, provided it has succeeded in reproducing and infecting new hosts.

How it ventures from host to host is unimportant as long as it is effective. Viruses are utilitarian, not averse to using transit when necessary. Both malaria and yellow fever are transmitted by mosquitoes, albeit different species. A mosquito that has bitten an infected person can then transfer the virus to a second individual it bites. The Black Death was initially brought to Europe by infected fleas riding on rats. When the fleas later jumped to human hosts they brought the virus with them. Microbial sources of pandemic – their myriad types, diverse methods of transmission and rapid mutation – are all simply fulfilling their biological imperative to survive long enough to reproduce.

There is a contrarian position that also needs to be borne in mind, that is in no way meant to minimise the individual suffering and death nor to compensate for the staggering death toll of pandemics: amid the nightmarish consequence, all pandemics tend to have at least some positive aftereffects; benefits for certain social classes and certain sectors of the economy. Even amid the horrors of COVID-19, it is impossible to deny the profound advantages for the environment. With air travel severely limited, industries shutting down and many commuters now working from home, air quality has improved substantially. Atmospheric emissions of everything from particulate matter to greenhouse gases have tumbled. Isaac Newton, socially distancing during the Great Plague of London, used his time productively to articulate the principles of calculus.

The situation of rural labourers improved in every sense after the Black Death since agricultural wages rose while rents fell. Labourers burdened by traditional liege obligations could simply walk away, as could indentured servants, and find work elsewhere. At the other end of the scale, wealthy victims of the plague left huge bequests that led to a burst of exceptional ecclesiastical and academic architecture. Cultural historians see the roots of the Florentine Renaissance in the psychic shock of the Black Death. Rarely does one hear the positive benefits of pandemics enumerated yet, as minimal as they may be, they are an integral part of the complete picture of life following a pandemic.

An accolade as unintended as it must be bitter, one of the big winners of the COVID-19 pandemic at the time of writing was Frank M. Snowden, Andrew Downey Orrick Professor Emeritus of History and History of Medicine at Yale University. Having spent 50 years in relative obscurity studying epidemics, primarily malaria and cholera in the nineteenth century, he published Epidemics and Society: From the Black Death to the Present in October 2019, only weeks before the emergence of COVID-19. At a door-stopping 600 plus pages, and a pocketbook breaking 60+ US dollars, released by an academic press, it has unexpectedly, but not surprisingly, become a bestseller.

In its introduction he makes plain the importance and impact of infectious diseases: "Epidemics are not an esoteric subfield for the interested specialist but instead are a major part of the 'big picture' of historical change and development. Infectious diseases, in other words, are as important to understanding societal development as economic crises, wars, revolutions, and demographic change." Orally, in the classroom, he is pithy, "Infectious diseases are too important to leave solely to the doctors." Combatting COVID-19 is the job of the doctors, analysing its future impact is the task of the book you are now reading; living with the aftermath will be the job of the survivors going forward.

Throughout, the focus will be on Europe and North America. This is solely a question of manageability. In reality, the regions outside of Europe and North America suffer epidemics more frequently and with greater loss of life. For the same reason, only selected epidemics will be considered. Those chosen, however, will be diverse: viral and bacterial, medieval and modern, wartime and peacetime.

It is essential, also, to realise that pandemics do not occur in an historical or social vacuum. The Spanish flu pandemic was preceded by the unprecedented cataclysm of the First World War. Inevitably, that influenced the epidemic. Most obviously, with the epidemic coinciding with the end of the war, demobilised soldiers, returning home, provided a perfect vector to spread the infection. However, there would also have been plenty of senseless suffering and death to go around in the war's wake even without the pandemic – which makes it difficult to tease out from the horrendous aftermath exactly what was a result of the pandemic and what was an inevitable consequence of the war. In sum, just because an event follows a pandemic does not necessarily mean it was a consequence of the pandemic.

Conversely, the Great Plague of London was immediately followed by a firestorm that gutted the heart of the city and destroyed 85% of its housing stock. Rebuilding, primarily with brick and stone rather than wood, is credited with saving London from both another Great Fire and another Great Plague. It is a considerable challenge to separate the consequences of the two cataclysms. The fire was blamed on foreign agents by some segments of the population and incidents of xenophobia were reported. To what extent this hysteria was exacerbated by the preceding epidemic is also a vexing issue.

Consider COVID-19 in the context of the geopolitical relationship between the People's Republic of China and the United States of America. Prior to the pandemic, the shifting power dynamic between the two existed and played a key role in global affairs. Arguably, it influenced both states' responses to the pandemic. China seems to have suppressed initial reports of the virus while the US placed too much emphasis on travel restrictions to and from China at the expense of other preparations. One of the key after effects of the COVID-19 pandemic will likely be its impact on this critical relationship. Pandemics, from the Black Death to COVID-19, occur in context. That tapestry of society and culture influences the whole timeline of a pandemic – from the initial response to the last of its aftershocks.

1.

Black Death

"What shall I say? How shall I begin? Whither shall I turn?
On all sides is sorrow; everywhere is fear.
I would, my brother, that I had never been born, or, at least,
had died before these times."

Francesco Petrarch, poet/humanist
He lost his Laura (d. 1348), his son, Giovanni (d. 1361),
and grandson, Francesco (d. 1368), to the bubonic plague

IN EUROPE, 1816 is known as 'The Year There was No Summer' and in New England it is remembered as 'Eighteen Hundred and Froze to Death.' Snow fell on Quebec City in the colony of Lower Canada, today the province of Quebec, in June. That same month, the Romantic poet Byron was hosting guests at Villa Diodati on Lake Geneva. Prevented by cold, wet, windy weather from enjoying the planned outdoor pursuits and trapped indoors the group was, unintentionally, socially isolating. To relieve the boredom, Byron challenged his guests to compose gothic tales of horror. Days later, on the night of June 16-17 [astronomers have confirmed the date based on a diary entry and the phases of the moon], one of his guests had the germ of an idea for a story entitled, 'The Modern

Prometheus'. That guest was Mary Shelley and the tale, the most widely recognised in the horror pantheon, known by the name of the monster's creator, is Frankenstein.

Almost five centuries earlier the Florentine scholar Giovanni Boccaccio set his work *The Decameron* in a country villa near Fiesole, on a hillside a short distance northeast of Florence. Ten friends tell tales to one another while socially distancing, sequestered from a terrifying plague ravaging Florence in 1348. Boccaccio, a sterner taskmaster than Byron, demands from each one tale every night for ten nights. Setting the stage, the framing story includes a gruesome description of the illness: "[T]here appeared certain tumors in the groin or under the arm-pits, some as big as a small apple, others as an egg; and afterwards purple spots in most parts of the body; in some cases large and but few in number, in others smaller and more numerous – both sorts the usual messengers of death."

This 14th century outbreak was the second great pandemic to sweep through Europe. The first had come in the middle of the 6th century, ravaging Constantinople and spread by ship around the coast of the Mediterranean. At its peak, 5000 people a day were dying in Constantinople, with the population ultimately halved. Overall, it is estimated that 25% of the Mediterranean world was wiped out in the first plague pandemic.

But that paled in comparison to the disease from which Boccaccio and his friends were sheltering – bubonic plague. It was highly infectious, virulent and killed its host quickly, features that made it all the more terrifying. It struck across all social classes, not preferentially targeting the poor, and attacked the hale and hearty as well as children and the elderly. It swiftly earned the sobriquet, 'the Black Death.'

The Black Death entered Europe aboard Genoese ships through Messina in Sicily and the ports of northern Italy. Florence was one of the first cities severely afflicted. Eventually, more than three-quarters of the population would die in one of Europe's first, and worst, hit cities.

Quantitatively and qualitatively it was the granddaddy of all pandemics. It killed a larger proportion of the European population than any other and had a more profound effect on society, culture and spirituality than any of the pandemic that followed. It also hung around for four centuries, recurring generation after generation. The last outbreak of the Black Death in Europe, bookending the first, also occurred in Messina, in 1743, 396 years after it first arrived there. For these reasons pandemic scholar Frank Snowden describes it as "the inescapable reference point in any discussion of infectious diseases and their impact on society … setting the standard by which other epidemics would be judged."

The origins of the bubonic plague, a disease caused by the bacterium *Yersinia pestis*, like much of the distant mirror that is the 14th century, are shrouded in myths buried under a misnomer. The bacteria is an eponym. It carries the surname of its discoverer, Alexandre Yersin – a dubious honour indeed. Contemporaries referred to the medical catastrophe it wrought as *atra mors*. The latter, meaning death, is evident in terms such as *rigor mortis* and mortuary. However, the first term, *atra*, has multiple meanings, including both black and terrible. Recent scholarship and textual analysis has reached a consensus that the reference is to the 'Terrible Death', not the 'Black Death'. Regardless, throughout, in the interests of convenience and convention, the events of 1346 to 1353 will be referred to as the Black Death. That said, contemporary references to 'the terrible death' speak to its psychological impact.

The Black Death's foundational myth requires more rigorous analysis. Its source is Gabriele de Mussi, a notary from Piacenza, north of Genoa. He described events in Kaffa (Feodosia), a Genoese trading outpost on the Black Sea coast of the Crimea when plague broke out in 1346 in *Istoria de Morbo sive Mortalitate quae fuit Anno Dni MCCCXLVIII* (*History of the Disease, OR The Great Dying of the Year of our Lord 1348*). At the time, the Crimea was part of the Golden Horde, the northwestern portion of the Mongol empire, and relations between the Genoese and the Mongols were terrible. Janibeg, the Khan, had besieged the colony since 1343. In 1344 an Italian relief expedition broke the siege and a year later an epidemic forced Janibeg to abandon his attempt to take the colony. In the winter of 1347-48, a second epidemic threatened yet another besieging force led by the Khan. De Mussi wrote, "But behold, the whole army was affected by a disease which overran the Tartars and killed thousands upon thousands every day. It was as though arrows were raining down from heaven to strike and crush the Tartars' arrogance." Arrows, the imagery of infection, and their origin, 'raining down from heaven', are both noteworthy.

This time, according to de Mussi, Janibeg took desperate measures and "ordered corpses to be placed in catapults [actually, trebuchet] and lobbed into the city in the hope that the intolerable stench would kill everyone inside." In one fell swoop he freed himself of the need to dispose of the bodies and infected the Genoese garrison. He is credited with the first use of biological weapons in recorded history.

According to *Guardian* contributor Simon Wessely, the incident never happened and de Mussi is guilty of hyperbole, "using the story as medieval tabloid journalism to illustrate Mongol frightfulness and corpse desecration." On the other hand, American microbiologist Mark Wheelis concludes the "theory is consistent with the technology of the times and with contemporary notions of disease causation." In other words it could be true. However, true or not, he goes on to declare it redundant; "the entry of plague into Europe from the Crimea likely occurred independent of this event." Simply put, it did not require airborne cadavers to infect the Genoese in Kaffa.

Kaffa was located near the Straits of Kerch between the Black Sea and the Sea of Azov. River boats bringing Oriental goods down the Don River from the Great Silk Road's terminus in central Russia would trade their goods in Kaffa. There, Genoese merchants would transfer the goods onto ships bound for Genoa and other European ports. Oriental rat flea (*Xenopsylla cheopis*) bearing black rats (*Rattus rattus*) would have accompanied the ships and goods. Above and beyond biological warfare, there were a multitude of connections between Europe and Asia via the Black Sea that would have transmitted the infection to Europe. While the precise methods of travel are unclear, the route is not. Bubonic plague travelled along the Great Silk Road from Asia into central Russia, down the Don River to Kaffa and thence onward to Europe.

Located on the Sea of Marmora between the Black and Mediterranean Seas, Constantinople was infected first, in the early summer of 1347. Messina, the seaport in Sicily, and the northern Italian ports followed. Simultaneously, the plague erupted in North Africa, at the Egyptian port of Alexandria. By the fall it had reached Marseilles, headed up the Rhône and crossed overland towards Bordeaux. The following spring, aboard a ship from Bordeaux it arrived in England at Weymouth and Bristol. By August 1348 it had reached

London and by the end of the summer had erupted in the northern port of Grimsby.

Initially, the bacterium *Yersinia pestis* was restricted to rats. Fleas that bite an infected rat become infected themselves. The bacteria eventually kills both. The bacteria kills by blocking the flea's gut; as the flea starves it embarks on a biting frenzy, sharing approximately 100,000 microbes per bite. Like the rabid dog, the bacteria actually alters the flea's behaviour to increase the likelihood of transmission. The rat population sickens and dies while the flea population increases. Ill rats, unable to groom themselves, become infested with increasing flea populations as death nears. When the rats die off, the fleas are forced to seek other hosts – humans.

When they bite their new hominid host they spread the infection. This also introduces a second vector. When a human (or house) flea (*Pulex irritans*) bites an infected human it too becomes infected and able to transmit the bacteria to other humans. The active maritime trade between the Black Sea and northern Italian ports meant that ships regularly made journeys back and forth. Aboard the ships, among the cargo, would have been infected rats and infesting those rats would have been infected fleas – all in close proximity to the crew. Rats and humans could not spread the bacteria, but the fleas they carried could. Fleas, infesting sailors, land and maritime traders and their goods, and rats, spread the Black Death.

The pace of the plague's march varied in direct proportion to the availability of transportation links and trade networks. In the countryside it advanced slowly, less than half a mile daily, basically from field to field among agricultural labourers. Along roads and between major towns it covered about 1.5 miles per day carried by traders and merchants themselves and among their goods. The spread by waterborne transport outpaced both of these routes. By sea it was intermittent, jumping from port to port and island to island, but could cover hundreds of miles in a fortnight. A healthy crew could board a ship carrying infected rats and sicken at sea. More than once, plague killed everyone on board before the vessel reached its destination. At the Black Death's height ghost ships drifted aimlessly on the Mediterranean Sea.

Links between Mediterranean traders and the Hanseatic League in northern Europe carried the plague into the Baltic Sea and Scandinavia. It leapt the English Channel. Along the great river systems of Europe and along the roads of the European trade network it spread inland. It travelled up the Danube and south on the Elbe into central Europe. From the North Sea, traffic on the Rhine carried it into the heart of western Europe and from the Mediterranean it spread into southern France along the Rhône. Ironically, Russia, a waystation on the disease's journey to Europe, was hit late – only when the plague advanced back east from Europe.

Arriving in Europe, *Yersinia petis* was venturing into virgin soil. Northern Europe had never seen the plague and Mediterranean Europe had not seen it since that initial 6th century outbreak. The population had no natural immunity, which meant the virus ran wild. Medical science, such as it was, could do nothing and there were minimal government institutions to standing ready to confront the disease. Generalised socio-economic decline further exacerbated the situation. An enduring recession and episodic famine characterised the entire first half of the 14th century and undermined overall health.

Torrential rains during the two years preceding the Black Death created a crisis. Flooded fields could not be planted and sodden fields could not be harvested. The dampness attenuated rinderpest (caused by the *morbillivirus*) which devastated livestock populations, killing draft animals and sources of meat and milk. (A few centuries earlier the *morbillivirus* mutated and, through a process called zoonosis, introduced its newfound human hosts to the disease we refer to as measles.) The burden was exacerbated by the response of the landholding nobility. Seeking to sustain their luxurious lifestyles, they increased rents and taxes, rigorously enforcing traditional *liege* obligations. *Yersinia pestis*, encountered a famished, enfeebled and unresisting host population when it arrived in 1347.

Before turning to the medical aspects of *Yersinia pestis*, it is necessary to confirm its identity. In his dotage, eminent Canadian-American medievalist Norman F Cantor published *In the Wake of the Plague*. An intriguing analysis of the consequences of the Black Death, it is prefaced by the bizarre argument that the Black Death was actually an anthrax pandemic. Suffice to say, Cantor was no microbiologist. And microbiologist Susan Scott is no zoologist. She argues that the Black Death could not have been bubonic plague because *Yersinia pestis* requires a particular species of rat, *Rattus rattus*, the black rat or ship's rat to reach pandemic levels in a human population. She concludes that since the black rat's range did not extend into northern Europe, neither could any disease it carried. However, Norwegian medievalist Ole Benedictow from the University of Oslo and a host of zoologists have placed *Rattus rattus* in Scandinavia well before the 14th century. Scott's assertion that the range of the black rat and of the Black Death must be coterminous is also wrong. If an infected person sailed from Genoa to London or up the Danube to Buda or Pest they presented no risk, but any fleas on them did.

When an infected flea bit a person there was typically a three to five day incubation period that was asymptomatic. The first symptoms appeared at the site of the bite; a purplish blister surrounded by a red ring. This telltale sign gave rise to the child's nursery rhyme, "Ring-a-ring o' roses,/A pocket full of posies,/A-tishoo! A-tishoo!/We all fall down." An aromatic 'pocketful of posies' was deemed protection from miasma – pestilential air – presumed to be the cause of the plague at the time. The infection was concentrated in the lymph nodes and this explains the characteristic hard purplish black buboes that developed as the infection progressed and the bacteria multiplied. A bite in the lower extremities caused buboes in the groin or on the thighs; a bite to the upper body led to buboes in the neck and armpit. Before this, the plague initially presented with flu-like symptoms – fever, chills, vomiting and fatigue.

According to friar Michele di Piazze, the infected, "were stricken with pains all over the body and felt a terrible lassitude. There then appeared, on a thigh or an arm, a pustule like a lentil." While the majority of the buboes may have been the size of a lentil, they could be as large as an orange. Michele di Piazze again: "Soon the boils grew to the size of a walnut, then to that of a hen's egg or a goose's egg, and they were exceedingly painful, and irritated the body, causing it to vomit blood by vitiating the juices. The blood rose from the affected lungs to the throat, producing a putrefying and ultimately decomposing effect on the whole body." A goose egg is typically three times the size of a hen's egg; di Piazze is referring to substantial buboes. He continues, "From this the infection penetrated the body and violent bloody vomiting began. It lasted for a period of three days and there was no way of preventing its ending in death."

The virus doubled in number every two hours and directly attacked the immune system. It targeted and killed white blood cells while also disabling the immune response. Reddish spots, known as 'tokens' appeared on the skin and fever rose. Untreated, the bacteria overwhelmed the immune system, poisoning the blood, causing septic shock. Throughout, the patient, their effusions and effluvia, all emitted a horrible stench. Eventually organ failure and neurological damage would kill.

Prior to death bubonic plague could develop into pneumonic or septicemic plague. The latter occurred when the virus entered the bloodstream from the lymphatic system, the former when it entered the respiratory system. Pneumonic plague, in the lungs, could be transmitted directly person to person via droplets expelled by coughing, sneezing, even talking, like COVID-19. At its peak, the plague could be transmitted by fleas *and* from person to person. It seems that this shift from bubonic to pneumonic plague occurred with increasing frequency over the four centuries that the disease lingered in Europe, but this transition always remained in the minority among cases.

The disgusting symptoms of the disease, its infectiousness and the sheer numbers of dead overwhelmed witnesses. Agnolo di Tura del Grasso manages to combine the personal and the public in an agonisingly touching recollection. "In many places in Siena great pits were dug and piled deep with the multitude of dead. And they died by the hundreds both day and night, and all were thrown in those ditches and covered over with earth. And as soon as those ditches were filled more were dug. And I, Agnolo di Tura, called the Fat, buried my five children with my own hands. And there were also those who were so sparsely covered with earth that the dogs dragged them forth and devoured many bodies throughout the city. There was no one who wept for any death, for all awaited death. And so many died that all believed that it was the end of the world." Di Tura was not alone in believing the apocalypse was upon him.

More than half of the population of Europe died of bubonic plague between 1347-1353. Benedictow concluded in 2005 that "the Black Death swept away around 60% of Europe's population. It is generally assumed that the size of Europe's population at the time was around 80 million. This implies that around 50 million people died in the Black Death." An equivalent mortality rate today would see 34 million deaths in England, 22.5 million deaths in Canada and 195 million in the USA. The death toll in Venice, Pisa, Florence and Genoa was estimated to be as high as 75%.

For the survivors, the social fabric had been shredded. The disease tore asunder bonds of friendship, even family. According to Boccaccio, "This tribulation pierced into the hearts of men, and with such dreadful terror that one brother forsook another, the uncle the nephew, the sister the brother, and the wife the husband. Nay, a matter much greater, and almost incredible: fathers and mothers fled away from their own children, even as if they no way appertained to them." Families abandoned infected members. Deaths overwhelmed the ability to bury the bodies. As noted earlier, the disease was so devastating because Europe was virgin territory; the population had no immunity because it had not encountered the microbe for centuries. People had no idea what was going on. Never before in living memory had such a tragedy befallen Europe.

The medieval mind had three paradigms that framed understanding of the plague: the medical or temporal, the celestial or astrological, and the divine. In *The Decameron*, Boccaccio notes some possibilities: "Some say that [the plague] descended upon the human race through the influence of the heavenly bodies, others that it was a punishment signifying God's righteous anger at our iniquitous way of life." He does not consider any earthly explanation worth mentioning.

Others speculated on a terrestrial event triggered by a celestial one. In France, the *Paris Consilium* was composed by the medical faculty at the University of Paris in October 1348, at the request of King Philip VI of France. It stated that the ultimate cause of the plague would never be known, that the truth was beyond human grasp, implying a divine origin. It did, however, offer a comprehensive explanation of the pandemic. It was recorded that, in 1345, "at one hour after noon on March 20, there was a major conjunction of three planets [Saturn, Mars and Jupiter] in Aquarius... Jupiter, being wet and hot, draws up evil vapors from the earth and Mars, because it is immoderately hot and dry, then ignites the vapors... This corrupted air, when breathed in, necessarily penetrates to the heart and corrupts the substance of the spirit there and rots the surrounding moisture, and the heat thus caused destroys the life force, and this is the immediate cause of the present epidemic."

This analysis combines two of the three paradigms: a celestial event, a planetary conjunction, triggers a miasma on earth "and this is the immediate cause of the present epidemic." The terrestrial cause was air poisoned with noxious gases released from the earth, commonly referred to for centuries as a miasma or miasmata. (The common name for the disease caused by the *Plasmodium* parasite – malaria – translates as *mal-* bad, *aria-* air, bad air.) This theory held sway for millennia and as 19th century cholera demonstrates in a later chapter, resisted displacement until the dawn of the 20th century despite a growing body of evidence to the contrary. It is for this reason – the behaviour of the air being key – that sanitary reports regularly commenced with meteorological details well into the 20th century. Medical theory held that when the poisoned air entered the body, it went to the heart, believed to be the organ of respiration, and imbalanced the humours. The Hippocratic text *Epidemics* stressed the importance of astrology and Aristotle's *Meteorology* linked increased 'putrefaction' to astrological phenomena. Suspected terrestrial sources of miasma included volcanoes, earthquakes, swamps, human and animal remains and waste, and other sources of disagreeable odours.

Regardless of the source, to the medieval mind it was clear that miasmata caused pandemic diseases. In the middle of the 14th century, tying the Black Death to a miasma linked to a celestial event was standard, widespread and commonly accepted. This misunderstanding of the disease rendered medical practitioners impotent. Debate focused on whether the astrological precursor was a cause of the miasmata or a warning of the catastrophe to come.

Practitioners' hands were tied too by the state of medical knowledge. The High Middle Ages placed great value on the classics in medical science. Consequently, medical knowledge was, literally, ancient. In the 14th century, physicians looked back to the second century CE Graeco-Roman physician Galen. He, in turn, cast his gaze back to a contemporary of Pericles and Thucydides, the Greek physician, Hippocrates. Hippocrates introduced the humoural theory of health. As incorrect as the theory was it was the first medical theory that proposed an alternative to a view that health and ill-health were simply a question of divine favour or disfavour. Hippocrates' theories definitely did not replace the theory of disease as divine judgement, as the Black Death demonstrates, but they did exist alongside it. Essentially, disease had a medical or physical cause but was, as were all things, ultimately, a manifestation of divine will and purpose.

Hippocratic medical theories, physical causes of health and illness, were based on the four humours, manifest as black and yellow bile, phlegm and blood. The physician did not treat a disease so much as he treated the body: illness was caused by humoural imbalance and the physician's objective was to tweak the patient's humours to restore balance and thereby good health. In *On the Nature of Man* Hippocrates wrote, "Health is primarily that state in which these constituent substances [the humours] are in the correct proportion to each other, both in strength and quantity, and are well mixed. Pain occurs when one of the substances presents either a deficiency or an excess, or is separated in the body and not mixed with others."

A pandemic, in this model, occurs when there is a widespread humoral imbalance. This is how they arrived at the theory of miasma, without understanding infection. If humoural imbalance was widespread, the cause had to be widespread, or possibly universal, and air fit the bill. It made intuitive sense that it was in the atmosphere. This misunderstanding rendered attempts to control the plague misdirected and, consequently, largely meaningless. As the Montpellier doctor Simon de Couvain lamented in 1350, the Black Death had left medicine in confusion; "the art of Hippocrates was lost".

This inability to cure the ill or stop the spread of the disease was coupled with an elevated death rate among doctors themselves as a consequence of their proximity to the sick. Together this led to widespread disdain for the calling and even attacks on practitioners. Medical geographer Peta Mitchell concludes, "Over the course of two millennia, then, the Hippocratic theory that disease was, at base, miasmatic in origin remained largely undisputed." And, unfortunately, wildly incorrect.

Doctors were stymied, unable to respond to the plague or halt the relentless march of death. The proposed treatments became increasingly bizarre and desperate. A group of doctors from Oxford recommended to the Lord Mayor of London, "If an ulcer appears... near the ear or the throat, take blood from the arm on that side, that is, from the vein between the thumb and the first finger... But if you have an ulcer in the groin, then open a vein in the foot between the big toe and its neighbour... At all events, bloodletting should be carried out when the plague first strikes." Venesection, or bleeding, was standard medical practice for centuries and widely prescribed for a host of ailments. It had no beneficial impact on plague victims.

The Lord Mayor also received instructions to prepare a treatment: "Take an egg that is newly laid, and make a hole in either end, and blow out all that is within. And lay it to the fire and let it roast till it may be ground to powder, but do not burn it. Then take a quantity of good treacle, and mix it with chives and good ale. And then make the sick drink it for three evenings and three mornings." Calcium, sugar and alcohol would have had just as little effect on the plague as bloodletting. Some posited that just looking at the infected was infectious and others argued that merely thinking about the disease caused it.

In the same vein, the PPE that medical practitioners wore was of little prophylactic value. A mask with an exaggerated beak filled with aromatic herbs and dried flowers and a droopy, wide brimmed hat protected the wearer from infectious miasma in the air. A waxed leather or canvas cloak completed the outfit, and may have provided some actual protection from picking up fleas. The staff that allowed them to examine patients, crudely, from a distance may also have offered some protection from the infected person's fleas. The relative uselessness of the doctor's distinctive costume illustrates their basic misunderstanding of the microbe they were dealing with. Nonetheless, the terrifying outfit would remain standard for centuries.

Although largely incomplete and ineffective, other measures to deal with pandemics that would become familiar over the coming centuries were introduced to deal with the Black Death. Despite gaping regional differences in their practices, ports usually made attempts to inspect and quarantine incoming ships and cargos. On land, *cordon sanitaire* of watchmen and constables were instituted, with varying success, to prevent people from entering and leaving infected districts. In a few cities health magistrates or nascent boards of health were equipped with emergency powers to enforce regulations in an attempt to restrict movement and improve sanitation and waste removal. However, government at all levels was miniscule by modern standards and virtually nonexistent at the municipal level.

All who could do so isolated themselves. The wealthiest abandoned the cities for their country villas in the manner of Boccaccio's narrators. As long as the miasma theory predominated, public health measures were largely sporadic and half-hearted – the only effective way to avoid the miasma was through flight. Smoky, sulphurous fires were burned to break up the miasma and for the same reasons cannon were fired. Pots were banged to make a racket because loud noises were thought to have a salutary effect on miasma – a tradition revived during this pandemic for different reasons.

On the deepest level, for the medieval psyche the plague was merely a proximate cause; a manifestation of something more profound. The essence of the experience was, as everything was for citizens of the 14th century, spiritual. The cataclysm was an instrument of God's wrath. The sheer scale of human loss was overwhelming. Death was so widespread that everyone was affected. Whole families vanished and cities were depopulated. Fields lay fallow, untended. Monasteries and convents were devastated. Everyone lost someone and according to pandemic historian Frank Snowden: "The result was not so much atheism as a mute despair that was most often barely articulated – a psychological shock that, with historical hindsight and anachronism, one might call posttraumatic stress." In the wake of the Black Death, Europe was reeling, punch drunk and staggering. Even Petrarch saw the plague as a divine judgement, "We have, indeed, deserved these [punishments] and even greater."

The idea that plague was a divine judgement was given weight by the simple fact that it killed an inordinately large number of ecclesiastics. Local priests had close contact with the infected, particularly administering last rites, and were often close to the dead and their fleas, looking for a new host as the deceased cooled. Professor Adrian R. Bell, a financial historian at Henley Business School in Buckinghamshire, UK, notes that Catholic priests were 'frontline workers' in medieval Europe. "In the 14th century there was a big demand for priests. Everyone who was dying had to be given the last rites, which meant the death toll among priests was huge and it is likely they had to fast-track replacements." The general population could not help but note the elevated fatality rate among priests.

The situation was even more problematic in monasteries, convents and other religious communities. These institutions often hosted fairs and markets and functioned as waystations for traders, their goods, rats and fleas. An infection would quickly kill the rat population and drive the fleas onto clerical hosts: Hosts who worshiped, worked and ate communally. Typical was the experience of Petrach's brother, Gherado, the lone survivor of 35 residents at his Carthusian monastery. In Aragon, 75% of the Dominican Order of Preachers active during 1348 were dead by 1351.

The Bible contains numerous tales of plagues and pestilence destroying the disobedient and God's enemies. It opens with a plague of boils on the Egyptians as the Israelite slaves make a bid for freedom and wraps up with the seven plagues of the Book of Revelations, that reprises boils and carbuncles, and presages Armageddon. Helpfully, many thought the biblical Book of Jonah offered an answer if the plague was indeed divine judgement. Jonah prophesied the destruction of the city of Nineveh, causing "the king and his nobles" to decree, "Let neither man nor beast, herd nor flock, taste any thing: let them not feed, nor drink water: But let man and beast be covered with sackcloth, and cry mightily unto God: yea, let them turn every one from his evil way, and from the violence that is in their hands." God takes note of their contrition and changed behaviour. "And God saw their works, that they turned from their evil way; and God repented of the evil, that he had said that he would do unto them; and he did it not." Repentance, mourning for past sins and self-denial saved Nineveh and there were those who assumed that it would work again.

The Flagellants believed that they could impact the plague, divine retribution being the core issue, by manifesting humility and self denial *in extremis*, self flagellation. They took a vow to not speak to the opposite sex, bathe or change their clothes. Then, all the while whipping themselves with leather thongs tipped with iron and bleeding freely, most often in pairs, and in large processions, they undertook pilgrimages of either 33 (the years of Christ's life) or 40 (Christ's passion, the flood, Pentecost, *ad infinitum*) days. Robert of Avesbury (d. 1359), Keeper of the Registry of the Court of Canterbury described a huge mob of flagellants: "In 1349 over 600 men came to London from Flanders... Each wore a cap marked with a red cross in front and behind. Each had in his right hand a scourge with three nails. Each tail had a knot and through the middle of it there were sometimes sharp nails fixed. They marched naked in a file one behind the other and whipped themselves with these scourges on their naked bleeding bodies." Extreme, bloody and painful self-abnegation made sense if the 'Terrible Death' was divine punishment.

Consequently, communities welcomed the Flagellants with church bells ringing and crowds singing, hoping their presence would please God and ease the calamity. In fact, the devout wanderers, their unwashed bodies and dirty clothes offering a free ride to fleas, often infected their grateful hosts.

Religious or spiritual excess, although rarely this extreme, is a frequent consequence of pandemics and episodes like this will be repeated. When HIV/AIDS first appeared, more than one televangelist identified it as divine punishment and that was less than 50 years ago.

As is its wont, this extremism often had a darker side, in this case scapegoating of, and pogroms against, outsiders, namely the Jews. The worst occurred in Strasbourg, the principal city in Alsace, in 1349. The city's Jewish community of 2000 was accused of causing the pandemic by poisoning the wells and ordered to abjure their religion. One thousand complied, the remainder were taken to the city's Jewish cemetery and burned alive. An ordinance was then passed prohibiting Jews from entering the city. The violent and tragic incident did nothing to stop the spread of the plague.

The morbid obsession with death and the afterlife was perfectly captured in the emerging image of the Danse Macabre. The universality of death is personified in a skeleton, often draped in a robe, but the hood and scythe of the grim reaper are later additions. In art and literature death begins to be depicted as a skeleton dance partner, bidding all to join them.

Images of pageants and *masques* presented people from all stations and classes bargaining with, and ultimately losing to, death. Rulers are told their arms and authority are powerless:

"Emperor, your sword won't help you out
Sceptre and crown are worthless here
I've taken you by the hand
For you must come to my dance."

The peasantry are told a life of neverending toil is no defence:
"I had to work very much and very hard
The sweat was running down my skin
I'd like to escape death nonetheless
But here I won't have any luck"

In the wake of the Black Death, the Danse Macabre assured one and all, high and low, that death was omnipresent. Financially, the Black Death was a windfall for the church. Expenses plummeted as the number of clerics to be paid shrank, as did the numbers of poor requiring alms. On the other side of the ledger, income skyrocketed as the great dying led to a decided jump in bequests from the now dead devout. Jean Venette, a Carmelite friar, noted the role the pope played in this. "To the even greater benefit of the dying, Pope Clement VI through their confessors mercifully gave and granted absolution from penalty to the dying in many cities and fortified towns. Men died the more willingly for this and left many inheritances and temporal goods to churches and monastic orders, for in many cases they had seen their close heirs and children die before them." Mercy may have motivated the pope, but money was the consequence.

The result was a spate of church building and renovation. Canterbury Cathedral in England was renovated and virtually rebuilt over a period of 30 years, beginning in 1377. Construction of the magnificent, gothic Black Church in Brasov, Transylvania began in the early 1380s. In Milan, one of the worst hit cities, ground was broken for a new cathedral in 1386. Two years later work started on St Barbara's Church, now a UNESCO World Heritage Site in Kutna Hora, Czech Republic.

The Black Death enhanced the appeal of St Sebastian, a third century soldier martyred by Diocletian. He was reputed to have been tied to a stake and repeatedly shot with arrows, a common visual symbol for the plague's infectiousness. In the wake of the Black Death his fame spread far beyond Rome, the site of his martyrdom. St Roch, a pilgrim who abandoned his odyssey to Rome to tend to the sick during the Black Death, a decision that was to cost him his life, was fast-tracked to sainthood and soared in popularity. Psalm 91, was also heard frequently and would come to be known as the 'Plague Psalm': "I will say of the Lord, He is my refuge, and my fortress, my God, in him will I trust. Surely he shall deliver thee from the snare of the fowler, and from the noisome pestilence." For the devout anything that reinforced faith was grasped like a lifeline.

The various and diverse impacts that the Black Death had on religion and spirituality speak to the complicated sequelae of pandemics. While it had helped the church to grow immensely wealthy, the high fatality rate had also left it extremely short-handed, sparking a recruiting drive that inevitably lowered the quality and the motivation of novitiates. For many, such as the

Flagellants, faith grew stronger, yet for others, perhaps because of the indiscriminate nature of the plague, it began to diminish.

It is no coincidence that the Renaissance welled up first in Florence, one of the worst afflicted cities. The inexplicable and incomprehensible deaths of good people undermined simple faith, inspiring spiritual questioning and laying the foundation for the Italian Renaissance. Scholars surviving the Black Death in northern Italy turned to neither the bible nor astrology, dismissing the divine and cosmology in favour of the classics. For Boccaccio and Petrarch, inspiration and wisdom lay in Greek and Roman literature and art. It is impossible to draw a straight, monocausal line from the Black Death to the Renaissance. Yet it is also impossible to deny the connection. The Black Death shook the foundations of the late medieval Church and the faith of individual believers.

In international affairs the pandemic had two noteworthy impacts. It eliminated population pressure in Scandinavia and put an end to Viking expansion. The decline in demand for walrus ivory in Europe after the Black Death may also have played a role in the extinction of the Vikings' Greenland colony. Without venturing into counterfactual history it is only reasonable to assert that the history of northeastern North America would be considerably different if Scandinavian penetration had persisted aggressively throughout the Renaissance as opposed to evaporating.

The pandemic also forced a brief intermission a decade into the Hundred Years' War. Immediately prior to the Black Death, England was on a roll in its war with France. An English army landed on the Cotentin peninsula during the summer of 1346 and marched across France to within miles of Paris, wreaking havoc. Finally brought to battle at Crécy in northern France on August 26, English longbowmen slaughtered the French forces. A week later they besieged Calais and it surrendered the following summer. The French king Philip IV was losing the war and his supporters bridled at increased taxes and levies to fund new armies and campaigns. English plans to press this advantage were brought to a screeching halt and the French monarchy saved – by the Black Death.

Then, as now, the pandemic caused massive, immediate and unforeseen economic dislocation. Average annual global inflation between 1360 and 1460 slowed to just 0.65% compared with 1.58% between 1311 and 1359, according to historian Paul Schmelzing's study analysing eight centuries of interest rates, published by the Bank of England in January 2020. Prices increased at an exceptionally slow rate. At the same time there was a desperate shortage of rural labourers – too many had died of the plague. This led to competition for the available labour, forcing wages up. Schmelzing's science was witnessed first hand by the French poet Guillaume de Machaut (c.1300-77):

"For many have certainly
Heard it commonly said
How in one thousand three hundred and forty-nine
Out of one hundred there remained but nine
Thus it happened for lack of people
Many a splendid farm was left untilled
No one plowed the fields
Bound the cereals and took in the grapes
Some gave triple salary
But not for one denier was twenty (enough)
Since so many were dead..."

In the wake of the Black Death the labour shortage was so severe that no matter what the wages there were simply not even enough survivors to till the available land.

The English monarchy recognised this and responded with legal action to compel rural society and the agricultural economy to conform to pre-plague practices, regardless of the radically changed circumstances. Nowhere is this clearer than in the Statute of Labourers of 1351. Its opening sentence clearly links the new laws to the Black Death. "Because a great part of the people and especially of the workmen and servants has now died in that pestilence, some, seeing the straights of the masters and the scarcity of servants, are not willing to serve unless they receive excessive wages, and others, rather than through labour to gain their living, prefer to beg in idleness."

According to Dene of Rochester, even the clergy were demanding better pay: "Many chaplains and hired parish priests would not serve without excessive pay. The Bishop of Rochester [by a mandate of June 27, 1349, to the Archdeacon of Rochester], commanded these to serve at the same salaries, under pain of suspension and interdict. Moreover, many beneficed clergy, seeing that the number of their parishioners had been so diminished by the plague that they could not live upon such oblations as were left, deserted their benefices." Simply, a shortage of labourers was driving up wages everywhere.

The statute responded by introducing wage controls. "Let no one, moreover, pay or permit to be paid to any one more wages, livery, meed or salary than was customary… Likewise saddlers, skinners, white-tawers [a fine leatherworking craft], cordwainers, tailors, smiths, carpenters, masons, tilers, shipwrights, carters and all other artisans and labourers shall not take for their labour and handiwork more than what, in the places where they happen to labour, was customarily paid to such persons in the said twentieth year of the reign of King Edward III [1346]" And price controls, "Likewise let butchers, fishmongers, hostlers, brewers, bakers, pullers and all other vendors of any victuals, be bound to sell such victuals for a reasonable price." The last paragraph of the Statute of Labourers makes charity illegal to force able-bodied poor to work at wage labour, "And because many sound beggars do refuse to labour so long as they can live from begging alms, giving themselves up to idleness and sins, and, at times, to robbery and other crimes – let no one, under the aforesaid pain of imprisonment presume, under colour of piety or alms to give anything to such as can very well labour, or to cherish them in their sloth, so that thus they may be compelled to labour for the necessaries of life." The Statute of Labourers was a revealing, direct and simple attempt to turn the clock back to the last pre-plague year, 1346, and was rigorously enforced.

It was supplemented with other legislation designed to sustain pre-plague social structures. With burgeoning income, labourers and craftsmen had newfound purchasing power too. Some of it was expended on apparel, finery including ermine collars and expensive dyes, notably purple – outrageously expensive because it could only be produced from the mucous of sea snails at the time. They were dressing and appearing above their station, so Edward III ruled that no one was to dress above the standard for their socio-economic status and craft or trade, than had been customary before the plague. (In Venice the height of women's platform shoes was regulated to ensure pre-plague standards were not exceeded.) These crude attempts to reset the clock were doomed to failure and ultimately blew up in England in the Peasants' Revolt of 1381 led by Wat Tyler.

The *Chronicles* of Jean Froissart explains the roots of the rebels' resentment: "Never was any land or realm in such great danger as England at that time. It was because of the abundance and prosperity in which the common people then lived that this rebellion broke out... The evil-disposed in these districts began to rise, saying, they were too severely oppressed... [that their lords] treated them as beasts. This they would not longer bear, but had determined to be free, and if they laboured or did any other works for their lords, they would be paid for it." In medieval England agricultural labourers had a variety of non-financial obligations to their lords and landowners, ranging from customary labour to a share of their produce. Depopulation and labour shortages had introduced a new level of mobility into the labour market. If an agricultural labourer disliked his traditional terms of service he could simply walk away. Moreover, many desperate landowners were happy to skirt the law and offer higher wages to attract labourers. In 1381 the intransigence of the landed class, expressed in the Statute of Labourers, crashed into the unrecognisable labour market of the post-plague world. Ultimately, the rebellion was suppressed and its leaders executed, but its eruption is testimony to the economic aftershocks of the Black Death.

Economically, the plague-induced labour shortage had at least one positive impact. It inspired a drive for increased productivity that led to a host of technological innovations in the ensuing decades. These included the crank and connecting rod to convert circular into reciprocal motion, the nautical compass, firearms and the blast furnace to cast cannon. This wave of innovation culminated in the revolutionary Gutenberg printing press in 1450. The variety of aftereffects of a pandemic inevitably includes some benefits; the current improvement in air quality is a modern example. However, the upsides to pandemics are always few and far between.

Demanding labourers and craftsmen, devious landlords willing to skirt the laws to attract labourers, shortages of food and other critical goods, and the shattered psyche of the observers all contributed to a sense that the world had gone mad, and mean, in the wake of the Black Death. In Paris, Venette lamented a world turned for the worse in every way: "For men were more avaricious and grasping than before, even though they had far greater possessions. They were more covetous and disturbed each other more frequently with suits, brawls, disputes, and pleas. Nor by the mortality resulting from this terrible plague inflicted by God was peace between kings and lords established. On the contrary, the enemies of the king of France and of the church were stronger and wickeder than before and stirred up wars on sea and on land. Greater evils than before [spread] everywhere in the world."

Agnolo di Tura del Grasso in Siena agreed, "when the pestilence abated, all who survived gave themselves over to pleasures: monks, priests, nuns, and lay men and women all enjoyed themselves, and none worried about spending and gambling. And everyone thought himself rich because he had escaped and regained the world…" A year later he added, " After the great pestilence of the past year each person lived according to his own caprice, and everyone tended to seek pleasure in eating and drinking, hunting, catching birds and gaming."

Matteo Villani knew of that which he wrote. The Black Death killed his famous brother, Giovanni, in 1348. Matteo carried on his brother's *Nuova Cronica* (*New Chronicles*) of Florence, including a description of economic dislocation and social disintegration: "since men were few, and since, by hereditary succession, they abounded in earthly goods, they forgot the past as though it had never been, and gave themselves up to a more shameful and disordered life than they had led before… And the common folk, both men and women, by reason of the abundance and superfluity that they found, would no longer labour at their accustomed trades, but demanded the dearest and most delicate foods for their sustenance; and they married at their will, while children and common women clad themselves in all the fair and costly garments of the ladies dead by that horrible death."

Del Grasso lamented, "all money had fallen into the hands of nouveaux riches." The traumatising experience of the Black Death created a devil-may-care attitude and provided the means to so indulge. While reading these accounts of moral turpitude and conspicuous consumption some skepticism is merited, but the conclusion is inescapable. Either society was more debauched in the wake of the plague, or the chroniclers themselves were so psychically shattered that they perceived society to be more debauched. Both interpretations speak to the profound, traumatic stress that followed the Black Death.

Bubonic plague was not a one trick pony. The plague eventually caught up with Matteo Villani in 1363 and killed him. It struck Petrarch's circle three times, although it spared him. The Black Death shattered the social order. It shook the foundations of the established church. Economically it appeared to have turned the world upside down. It even impacted on fashion. The impacts were wide and varied, some subtle, some shocking. For almost 400 years it would be endemic in Europe, with periodic fierce explosions. More than three centuries later it would ravage London, slaughtering 100,000 people, one-quarter of the population of one of the largest cities in the world at the time.

2.

The Great Plague of London

"A plague is a formidable enemy,
and is arm'd with terrors,
that every man is not sufficiently fortified to resist,
or prepar'd to stand the shock against."

H. F., narrator of Daniel Defoe's,
A Journal of the Plague Year

L ONDON WAS well acquainted with *Yersinia pestis* long before the Great Plague of 1665. The city lost 30,000 people, one-tenth of its residents, to the plague in 1603, 35,000 in 1625, and another 10,000 in 1636.

During the decade that followed the severe epidemic of 1603, London theatres were closed almost two-thirds of the time to limit community spread. Shakespeare's creative burst during this period corresponds with the time that Globe theatre was closed and he was not obliged to act, direct and manage a theatre company. Some Shakespeareans have even suggested that the melancholy gloom pervading King Lear, was plague-related. It was written in the wake of the 1603 epidemic that claimed the life of the bard's landlady and dear friend Marie Mountjoy.

Excepting the Black Death, London was hit hardest by bubonic plague in 1665-66. Daniel Defoe's description of the buboes was no different than those of 300 years earlier, "those spots they called the tokens were really gangrene spots, or mortified flesh in small knobs as broad as a little silver penny, and hard as a piece of callous or horn." In 18 months it killed upwards of 100,000, 25% of the population in one of the world's largest cities, fast becoming the heart of a global empire. It was the last time that bubonic plague would erupt in England and by then Londoners and their leaders were familiar with it. Although they understood plague little better in medical terms than they did centuries earlier, they had practical experience and standard operating procedures – one of which was documentation.

Bills of Mortality, a statistical accounting of all deaths in and around the city sorted by parish and cause of death were published weekly providing valuable granular data and often intimate details of the deceased. Unfortunately, the fire a year after the pandemic consumed many churches and parish records are incomplete and spotty. There exist also a variety of publications for medical practitioners and the general public offering both preventatives and treatments. Two widely known sources are invaluable: the personal diary of Admiralty official Samuel Pepys (pronounced Peeps) and an account, presented as fiction, by writer Daniel Defoe who was only a child during the events he describes in *A Journal of the Plague Year*. However, he had the benefit of his father's and his uncle's recollections as well as making an extensive investigation of the parish records and London government documents.

Samuel Pepys was born in London in 1633, a generation before Defoe. His father was a tailor and his mother the daughter of a butcher, mistakenly leading to the assumption that he rose from the lower classes. In fact, his father's will attests to a significant estate. Pepys's Cambridge education was partially funded by the Worshipful Company of Mercers (Merchants), the oldest and most influential of the London guilds. His great uncle, Richard Pepys, had been Chief Justice of Ireland from 1654 until his death in 1659. Most importantly, his patron during the epidemic was no lesser a personage than the Earl of Sandwich, Edward Montague (d. 1672). Montague's mother, Paulina Pepys (d. 1638) of Cottenham, was Samuel Pepys great aunt, making the Earl his second cousin. In the diary, Pepys worries about his patron's place in the pecking order that was the intrigue of the Restoration court more often than he documents his own internecine struggles.

The Earl of Sandwich played a key role in the restoration of Charles II in 1660, and while remaining a fighting admiral he was promoted to First Lord of the Admiralty. At the time, Pepys moved from the Earl's household staff to the Admiralty. When plague broke out in 1665 the Royal Court and much of the naval bureaucracy fled the city. Having just celebrated his 32nd birthday, Pepys remained in London, and with England at war with the Dutch he was incredibly busy and, operating in a near vacuum, influential. As he put it at the height of the epidemic, "the infinite business of the office, and nobody here to look after it but myself."

His observations on the plague alternate with details of the amorous adventures of himself and others, war news, ongoing attempts to manage the recently obtained, expensive and short-lived English colony of Tangier on the Barbary Coast, and efforts to negotiate loans for the king from the City of London and local notables. In pursuit of the latter he visits recently knighted banker Sir Robert Viner at Swackeley House, giving rise to surely his most bizarre diary entry, "He showed me a black boy that he had, that died of a consumption, and being dead, he caused him to be dried in an oven, and lies there entire in a box."

The veracity of his observations in the diary are attested to by an unusual, but unimpeachable source, himself. Pepys is painfully honest about his short-comings. He confesses to pursuing younger women, he particularly had an eye for actresses, often over drinking and to the remorse and regret that followed. This honesty is taken as evidence that the diary was never intended for publication or to polish his image. Many published diaries are altered and redacted prior to publication, by the memoirist or his allies, but this does not seem to be the case with Pepys.

Events elsewhere continued to unfold even as epidemic grew in London. The Second Anglo-Dutch War erupted at the same time as the plague outbreak. As London's death toll climbed, in June 1665, the Dutch suffered the worst defeat in the history of the Dutch Republic's navy, with at least 16 ships lost, and one-third of its personnel killed or captured at the battle of Lowestoft. The next day, before news of the battle had reached London, June 14, Pepys noted in his diary, "The town grows very sickly, and people to be afraid of it; there dying this last week of the plague 112, from 43 the week before." When he did hear news of the Dutch defeat on Tuesday, the 16th, the plague faded into the background as he gloried in the victory. However, his foremost concern was for his mentor's role and reputation: "My Lord Sandwich, both in his councils and personal service, hath done most honourably and serviceably." His honest admission of both patriotism and personal interest stands as testimony to the diary's candour, as does his foppish obsession with fashion, even amidst the devastation.

On the last day of July 1665, with the plague settled over London and another major sea battle with the Dutch impending, he attended a marriage he had helped to arrange. Too late for the ceremony, he met the wedding party returning from the church, and joined the festivities, taking care to note his finery, "I being in my new coloured silk suit, and coat trimmed with gold buttons and gold broad lace round my hands, very rich and fine." One month later he delights in wearing a new hairpiece while worrying about its post-plague future: "Sept. 3, 1665 (Lord's day). Up; and put on my coloured silk suit very fine, and my new periwig... and it is a wonder what will be the fashion after the plague is done, as to periwigs, for nobody will dare to buy any hair, for fear of the infection, that it had been cut off the heads of people dead of the plague." Pandemics often have a significant impact on insignificant habits. It is not without precedent that COVID-19 may spell the death of the handshake.

Daniel Defoe is recognised as one of the first English novelists and his most famous, *Robinson Crusoe* (1719), is reputed to be the most translated book in the world after the Bible. *A Journal of the Plague Year*, despite the title, is not a spontaneous personal journal of events as they occurred, but rather creative nonfiction, a historical record of the pandemic, presented as a novel. Defoe (born Daniel Foe) had just turned five when the plague struck London. His father, James, was a prosperous tallow chandler (candle maker) whose brother, Henry, was a London saddler (a craftsman producing leather accoutrements for horses, hansom cabs and carriages). Both men's trades forced them to remain in London during the plague and it is assumed that the *Journal* is largely built around their recollections. Indeed, it is undersigned, 'H. F.' (presumably, Henry Foe).

These reminiscences were supplemented by Defoe's research into primary sources, notably parish records that offered data on individual neighbourhoods. It shares with the *Diary* a deft combination of impartial documentation of the plague's progress, geographically and chronologically, with a compassionate eye for the individual suffering of tens of thousands of innocent victims; both the dead and the dazed, grieving survivors. The authors' attempts to maintain their own safety, and their chronicling of attempts by authorities and medical practitioners to constrain the plague, illustrate what was, and was not, learned about *Yersini pestis* over the four centuries it stalked Europe.

Defoe was dealing with a dangerous subject, bubonic plague, in a very topical work. The *Journal* was written and published in 1721, while a bubonic plague epidemic was in the process of killing tens of thousands in Marseilles. Its reoccurrence in London was a very real possibility at the time and the Great Plague was a scant half-century in the past. In this sense the *Journal*, intended as a warning, offers a timeline as an outbreak of bubonic plague erupts and explodes into a raging epidemic. It is driven by a sense of impending doom, a journal of a pandemic foretold. Pepys's diary has the advantage of immediacy, his shock and awe as the death count multiplies to unimaginable levels is recounted daily and is unfiltered.

There is a third volume, less known than these two, that is even more interesting. It is a second work of Defoe's, written at the same time as the *Journal*; a self-help book called *Due Preparations for the Plague, as Well for Soul as Body*. Defoe was hoping to spur England's government and governed into preparing to deal with the plague should it travel from Marseilles. According to Defoe, bodily preparations should include personal and community measures taken *before* the arrival of a pandemic. Preparations for the soul focused on spiritual (read psychological) preparations for isolation and death *during* a pandemic because plague is a physical health and a mental health threat: "A plague is a formidable enemy, and is armed with terrors, that every man is not sufficiently fortified to resist, or prepared to stand the shock against." Defoe wrote the *Journal* to capitalise on his success with *Robinson Crusoe* (published three years earlier) and to popularise the preventative measures laid out in *Due Preparations*. Both of Defoe's plague volumes were written to address a clear and present danger, influence public policy and increase popular awareness of the threat of plague.

There were minimal advances in medical science between the Great Plague of London in 1665-66 and *Due Preparations'* publication half a century later and it provides a valuable guide to the plague countermeasures of the time, particularly when supplemented by other medical texts from the 17th century. *Due Preparations* describes individual (or household) responses such as stockpiling foodstuffs and limiting travel and contact as 'particular measures'. "General, Public and National Preparations" include "measures which Government or magistrates may take to preserve the people from infection... To limit and prohibit commerce with places infected, and restrain the importation of such goods as are subject to be infected." He also advocates the French methods (aka *cordon sanitaire*), "surrounding the towns where it shall happen to be with troops of soldiers, cutting off all communication." However, he laments that as with smuggling, troops can be avoided, while the healthy trapped with the sick will struggle mightily to avoid the pickets and escape the quarantine area. Furthermore, entrepreneur first and author second, he argues that quarantine, "would be such a general interruption of trade, that it would entirely ruin the countries and towns so cut off, and the people would be very tumultuous and uneasy upon that head." He prefers the method also adopted in 1665-66, the locking down of individual houses if they become infected.

He regards quarantining communities as a last resort and proceeds to outline an entirely impractical system. In order to prevent the healthy being interned with the infected, he insists that all asymptomatic individuals be removed from a community about to be quarantined at the last moment and relocated. Such a measure would release many asymptomatic but infected individuals into surrounding communities and contribute to transmission. Regardless, his aversion to quarantine, *cordon sanitaire* and other restrictions on the movement of individuals and goods is ultimately predicated on his commercial priorities. Competition between public health measures and the demands of the economy are hardly unique to the current pandemic.

Government power had practical limits in the 1660s. Defoe notes this in *Due Preparations* with reference to trade barriers being constantly avoided by smugglers in normal times and only more so, and more dangerously, in times of plague, when "it is the worst sort of murder" to bring an infection into the country with smuggled goods. He also concedes that the government is ill-equipped to prevent it, "It is confessed that this is a difficulty even to the government itself, and it will be hard to say what they can do more than is done effectually to prevent this dreadful trade." England had only a small standing army to enforce *cordon sanitaire* and the navy was occupied elsewhere, warring with the Dutch.

The king and the national government were constrained further by specific circumstances. The Houses of Parliament, as we shall see, were paralysed due to relocation and Charles II, the 'Merry King', had little authority and even less desire to rule. He had been acceptable as the restoration monarch because he had more interest in the trappings of power than power itself. Further, he was broke. He desperately needed money from the city and its wealthiest residents. The national government was largely on the sidelines during the epidemic and authority would devolve onto the nascent municipal government.

Defoe was a confirmed miasmatist, but he did not believe in a generalised or universal contamination of the air. He believed offal, swamps and other odourous locations could produce plague but he also believed that the emanations of the sick polluted the air around them, creating an infectious cloud. "The effluvia of infected bodies may, and must be indeed conveyed from one to another by air… But those effluvias cannot extend themselves a great way, but, like ill smells, as they spread they die in the air, or ascend and separate, lose themselves, and are rarefied in the air, so as to lose all their noxious or infectious quality." Pepys took note that pedestrians took to the middle of the empty streets to avoid, "Smells and scents from houses that might be infected." Right theory for a respiratory virus (like COVID-19), but wrong disease. Bubonic plague was still, of course, relying on rats and fleas for transmission, so proximity to the ill and their infected fleas was a risk, but it had little to do with airborne droplet transmission barring cases that had become pneumonic.

Miasmatic theories led Dafoe to accept flight as the first response to the disease. In the second week of June the plague emerged within the city proper, that is within the historic Roman walls. But to Defoe the most noteworthy occurrences of the month were the realisation among the upper classes that the plague had indeed arrived and their subsequent flight. "The richer sort of people, especially the nobility and gentry, from the west part of the city thronged out of town, with their families and servants in an unusual manner… Indeed nothing was to be seen but wagons and carts, with goods, women, servants, children, etc. Coaches filled with people of the better sort, and horsemen attending them, and all hurrying away." This can be clearly recognised as social isolation; those who had country houses were fleeing, with their valuables and household staff. The rush was occasioned by rumours that travel would be prohibited and flight might soon be impossible. The best advice from the narrator's brother regarding the plague concurs: "run away from it." Later, he repeats, "it is my opinion, and I must leave it as a prescription, (viz.) *that the best physick against the plague is to run away from it.* [emphasis in the original]" This desire to flee to country estates, lakeside cottages, rural retreats and gated communities has also been evident in the current pandemic.

Parliament moved north, sitting in Oxford. The king and the entire court took to the road. Initially, they removed themselves to Hampton Court, then on to Salisbury. When a court groom became infected at Salisbury, the royal party headed north to Milton, just south of Oxford. According to H. F., "Great numbers of persons followed the court, by the necessity of their employments, and other dependencies: and as others retired, really frighted with the distemper." Those that could, some captains, sailors, watermen, merchants and their families, moved onto ships in the Thames and self-isolated afloat. "As the richer sort got into ships, so the lower rank got into hoys, smacks, lighters and fishing-boats; and many, especially watermen, lay in their boats." King Charles II and the court would not return to London until February of the following year.

While parliament fled and the court ambled about the countryside, the London city government took the opposite approach and publicly proclaimed that they were going nowhere. Unlike the royal court, the mayor and aldermen of London were determined to stay and confront the plague. According to H. F., they publicly announced "That they would not quit the city themselves, but that they would be always at hand for the preserving good order in every place, and for the doing justice on all occasions; as also for the distributing the public charity to the poor; and in a word, for the doing the duty, and discharging the trust reposed in them by the citizens to the utmost of their power." Defoe's narrator is full of praise for them: "Likewise the proper officers, called my Lord Mayor's officers, constantly attended in their turns, as they were in waiting... In like manner the sheriffs and aldermen did in their several stations and wards, where they were placed by office; and the sheriff's officers or sergeants were appointed to receive orders from the respective aldermen in their turn; so that justice was executed in all cases without interruption." The city government would prove to be the most important level of government in responding to the pandemic.

Defoe's epidemiological ignorance was hardly uncommon and indicates how impoverished medical knowledge remained. Arguably, his preceding theorising was on a certain level above that of other medical practitioners as the following list of proposed preventative and therapeutic concoctions demonstrates. Wearing arsenic in an amulet around the neck was advocated as a preventative. Another concoction included almost a pound of unicorn horn. Syphilis was said to deliver immunity to the plague. Laudanum, opium dissolved in brandy, was a popular prescription that would certainly have made the patient feel better although Defoe's narrator was opposed to excessive alcohol consumption. "Neither did I do, what I know some did, keep the spirits always high and hot with cordials, and wine, and such things, and which, as I observed, one learned physician used himself so much to, as that he could not leave them off when the Infection was quite gone, and so became a sot for all his life after."

For his part the narrator swears by Venice treacle, "I several times took Venice treacle, and a sound sweat upon it, and thought myself as well fortified against the Infection as any one could be fortified by the power of physic." Venice treacle is a classical mixture of 64 ingredients including plant and animal parts, minerals, oils and resins rendered palatable by honey according to the *Amsterdammer Apotheek* (1683).

The failure of medical practitioners, their impotence in the face of the infection, was obvious. "The plague defied all medicines; the very physicians were seized with it, with their preservatives in their mouths; and men went about prescribing to others and telling them what to do, till the tokens were upon them, and they dropt down dead, destroyed by that very enemy, they directed others to oppose." The failure of the professional provided fertile ground for the quacks and charlatans that H. F. disdains. "With what blind, absurd and ridiculous stuff, these oracles of the devil pleased and satisfied the people, I really know not; but certain it is, that innumerable attendants crowded about their doors every day." They offered cures which at best did nothing, and at worst killed those taking them – many containing poisonous mercury and other toxic ingredients.

Recognised medical practitioners and mountebanks alike were unable to protect themselves, let alone their patients. The medical treatment of the buboes was particularly gruesome, "Nay there was another thing which made the mere catching of the distemper frightful, and that was the terrible burning of the caustics, which the surgeons laid on the swellings to bring them to break, and to run." In terms of humoural medicine the procedure made sense. The body was attempting to expel a humour in excess to restore balance and the physician was facilitating that natural process. In fact, it did nothing but add another layer of agony to the diseased.

The first plague deaths were recorded at the north end of Drury Lane, just west of St Giles in the Fields, in April. Initially, optimists insisted it was not plague. However, according to Defoe's narrator the powers that be were aware of the situation and covering it up. "But it seems that the Government had a true account of it, and several counsels were held about ways to prevent its coming over; but all was kept very private. Hence it was, that this rumour died off again, and people began to forget it, as a thing we were very little concerned in, and that we hoped was not true." Again, the very same has been said about many governments during this crisis.

By mid-June, as the wealthy fled, the truth could no longer be denied; "the Parish of St Giles's, where still the weight of the infection lay, buried 120, whereof though the bills said but 68 of the plague; everybody said there had been 100 at least, calculating it from the usual number of funerals in that parish as above," according to Defoe's narrator. Six months earlier, the weekly mortality rate in the parish had averaged 15, meaning 'everybody' was probably correct when they placed plague deaths at 100 per week, and, overall the mortality rate had increased eightfold. Clearly the reputation of St Giles for being the most infected parish in the city and its environs was something that officials were willing to lie to avoid confirming. The approach and arrival of the plague had been downplayed, and now local officials were fudging the record to disguise its severity. Pandemics often inspire official falsehoods or obfuscation. During the current pandemic, the government of the Canadian province of Ontario has resisted making public granular data on infections claiming it would stigmatise the worst afflicted neighbourhoods and communities and refused to name the epidemiologists and scientists advising them on plague responses. Both the quality of government messaging and the accuracy and relevance of official statistics were contentious issues long before this most recent pandemic.

St Giles was only one of London's more than 100 parishes at the time. It was outside the old city walls, to the northwest, one of the crowded, sprawling suburbs that housed the tradesmen, craftsmen and household staff that serviced the city. In the words of Defoe's narrator, "in the out-parishes, which being very populous, and fuller also of poor, the distemper found more to prey upon than in the city." It would become one of the worst hit neighbourhoods in the London metropolitan area with the monthly death toll topping 1000.

The death toll was so high that it, literally, shook the church to its very foundation. A huge numbers of bodies from the neighbourhood were buried in the churchyard; eventually hundreds were crammed in helter skelter, even in ditches and mass graves. So many, in fact, that by 1711 the quantity of earth displaced and the decomposition of the bodies replacing it had caused the church's foundation to fail, threatening the entire structure. Gravity exerts downward force on a foundation. However, some of this is translated into lateral, outward force by the triangularity of the rafters of the roof. Rubble foundations, as opposed to modern reinforced concrete foundations, are particularly prone to this type of failure. As the bodies in the churchyard decayed and lost volume, the foundation's ability to resist lateral force declined. The foundation bowed, reducing its height, causing the walls above to subside. The parish applied for funds to restore the church under the New Churches in London and Westminster Act 1710, a belated response to the fire of 1666 designed to see 50 churches built. Initially, the application was declined as the Commission deemed that the restoration of an existing church was not a new construction, despite the plans requiring and including an entirely rebuilt foundation. Eventually, the decision was overturned and £8000 was granted. A new church was built between 1730 and 1734.

In contrast Samuel Pepys's own church, St Olave's, where he worshipped and is interred, had quite a different problem. So many bodies had been shallowly buried and then covered in soil that the churchyard was four feet higher than it had been pre-plague. The church's brand spanking new (1658) entranceway, that is famously decorated with miniature daemonic heads, was now below grade and a wide stone staircase had to be constructed *down* to it.

When one considers the demands placed on churchyards these bizarre consequences are not entirely surprising. Defoe's narrator describes the burials in the churchyard of his parish, Algate, as the plague took hold: A pit, "near as I may judge, it was about 40ft in length, and about 15 or 16ft broad; and at the time I first looked at it, about 9ft deep; but it was said, they dug it near 20ft deep afterwards, in one part of it, till they could go no deeper for the water." Two weeks later it was full, holding 1114 bodies dead of the plague.

The Lord Mayor had ordered that burials were only to occur from sunset to sunrise, to minimise the impact of the procession of 'dead-carts'. Defoe's narrator describes an encounter, "The cart had in it 16 or 17 bodies, some were wrapped in linen sheets, some in rugs, some little other than naked, or so loose, that what covering they had, fell from them, in the shooting out of the cart, and they fell quite naked among the rest; but the matter was not much to them, or the Indecency much to any one else, seeing they were all dead, and were huddled together into the common grave of mankind."

Pepys had a similarly ghoulish nocturnal encounter in the blackness of a new moon on August 15, 1665: "It was dark before I could get home, and so land at Church-yard stairs, where, to my great trouble, I met a dead corpse of the plague, in the narrow ally just bringing down a little pair of stairs. But I thank God I was not much disturbed at it. However, I shall beware of being late abroad again." A policy of only nighttime burials was eventually defeated by volume and burials occurred around the clock. For the same reason, sheer numbers led churches to stop tolling their bells for funerals.

Death and internment, one of the most solemn and intimate rituals in all cultures, overwhelmed by quantity, became a utilitarian, volume-oriented task. "The funerals became so many, that people could not toll the bell, mourn, or weep, or wear black for one another, as they did before; no, nor so much as make coffins for those that died," H. F. laments.

For those unable to flee, but with enough money to hoard, self isolation and social distancing were options: "Many families foreseeing the approach of the distemper, laid up stores of provisions, sufficient for their whole families, and shut themselves up, and that so entirely, that they were neither seen or heard of, till the Infection was quite ceased, and then came abroad sound and well." In *Due Preparations*, Defoe devotes considerable space to a meticulous list of everything that a wealthy family needs to acquire to socially isolate. Defoe's narrator has a positive view of hoarding and laments that he started doing it so late in the game. He also recognises the burden daily shopping placed on the poor and household staff: "However, the poor people could not lay up provisions, and there was a necessity, that they must go to market to buy, and others to send servants or their children; and as this was a necessity which renewed itself daily; it brought abundance of unsound people to the markets, and a great many that went thither sound, brought death home with them. One approach was to try to shut out the plague." Poverty forced the poor into the public marketplace frequently, risking being infected or infecting others, another hole in any system of quarantine or isolation.

With the wealthiest fleeing and those who could afford to hoarding and shutting themselves up in their homes, Pepys documents a previously bustling metropolis shutting down. In July he notes, "by coach home, not meeting with but two coaches, and but two carts from White Hall to my own house, that I could observe; and the streets mighty thin of people. In August, "two shops in three, if not more, generally shut up," and a month later he somberly noted, "To Lambeth. But, Lord! what a sad time it is to see no boats upon the river; and grass grows all up and down White Hall court, and nobody but poor wretches in the streets!" A city that had once teemed with people, with hansom cabs, carriages and carts, had gone silent, its streets slowly growing over.

Amid the silence of a shuttered city H. F. recalls the 'plague psalm', Psalm 91: "I will say of the Lord, He is my refuge, and my fortress, my God, in him will I trust. Surely he shall deliver thee from the snare of the fowler, and from the noisome pestilence." In doing so he was invoking spiritual inspiration that had fortified plague victims for centuries. He concludes that if it is God's will he perish, he will, whether he is in London or Lincolnshire, and resolves to stay put. He dismisses the astrologers' insistence that the appearance of a comet had foretold the disaster, although he notes that the theory had purchase with the population at large. Like the Flagellants and his plague predecessors, however, he does recall Jonah and his warning to the sinful, but saved, city of Nineveh.

Defoe's narrator believes there are terrestrial means that cause and spread plague somehow associated with air or miasma. But regardless, he remains convinced that the pandemic is fundamentally divine judgement: "As the divine power has formed the whole scheme of nature, and maintains nature in its course; so the same power thinks fit to let his own actings with men, whether of mercy or judgment, to go on in the ordinary course of natural causes, and he is pleased to act by those natural causes as the ordinary means." In other words, the pandemic has physical means of transmission and vectors of infection, but the manifestation of this infection is, ultimately, an expression of divine displeasure.

This being the case, a spiritual response was entirely appropriate and Pepys records a day of fasting on July 12, 1665 "A solemn fast-day; for the plague growing upon us." This approach is epitomised by *Due Preparations* which devotes its largest attention to spiritual preparations for plague. The plague also brought forth religious extremism and apocalyptic preachers. Defoe's narrator remarks on one Solomon Eccles, aka Solomon Eagle, a fanatical Quaker, "I suppose the world has heard of the famous Solomon Eagle an enthusiast: He tho' not infected at all, but in his head; went about denouncing of judgment upon the city in a frightful manner; sometimes quite naked, and with a pan of burning charcoal on his head." Defoe considered a spiritual response to plague appropriate, even viewing it as divine judgement, but he was neither an extremist nor a fanatic. Nor was Solomon Eagle a Flagellant although one wonders how he crowned his outfit, or lack thereof, with 'a pan of burning charcoal' without some discomfort.

While plague expressed divine judgement it had earthly causes and so too, over three centuries, terrestrial preventatives had been developed. On July 1, 1665 the city government acted decisively, publishing, "Orders Conceived and Published by the Lord Mayor and Aldermen of the City of London, concerning the Infection of the Plague. 1665." The Lord Mayor's Orders outline the standard operating procedures or best practices for a city confronting the plague at the time.

They decreed that parishes appoint examiners to seek out those infected so parish constables could 'shut up' houses of infected individuals for 28 days and appoint watchmen to prevent access and egress. By shut up was meant bolted and locked up, with the inhabitants, healthy and infected, inside. It was frequently a death sentence for both. Locksmiths and blacksmiths were as overworked as grave diggers and coffin makers. The rate to seal a door was three shillings and tuppence. The parish was expected to provide provisions, but often their social services were overwhelmed by numbers.

The minds of the 'locked up' apparently also worked overtime. Defoe devotes endless paragraphs to the ingenious methods they devised to circumvent being locked up. They ranged from the venal – bribing the watchman – through the mechanical – picking the lock and tampering with the bars and hasps – to the gymnastic – leaping across rooftops to a dwelling not locked up. Pepys relates a similar incident: "Mr Marr telling me by the way how a maid-servant of Mr John Wright's (who lives thereabouts) falling sick of the plague, she was removed to an out-house, and a nurse appointed to look to her; who, being once absent, the maid got out of the house at the window, and run away."

In September he complained, "there being now no observation of shutting up of houses infected, that to be sure we do converse and meet with people that have the plague upon them." Then as now, constraints on individual behaviour, no matter how justified or necessary, inspired noncompliance. Consequently, Defoe's narrator, believes the policy was a failure, "the setting of watchmen thus to keep the people in, was (first) of all, not effectual, but that the people broke out, whether by force or by stratagem, even almost as often as they pleased." As noted earlier, Pepys concurred. The city was attempting to apply quarantine measures but stumbling in the execution.

The orders also shuttered gathering places. "All plays, bear-baitings, games, singing of ballads, buckler-play [an action-drama with lots of swordplay as in swashbuckler] or such like causes of assemblies of people, be utterly prohibited… All public feasting, and particularly by the companies of this city, and dinners at taverns, alehouses, and other places of common entertainment be forborne till further order and allowance." Schools, from grammar to dancing and fencing, were closed. Finally, "disorderly tippling in taverns, alehouses, coffee houses, and cellars be severely looked unto, as the common sin of this time, and greatest occasion of dispersing the plague." Restricting public gatherings and quarantine are still being employed today, 350 years later.

The Lord Mayor's Orders also addressed vagrancy. "The multitude of rogues and wandering beggars, that swarm in every place about the city, being a great cause of the spreading of the Infection… no wandering beggar be suffered in the streets of this city, in any fashion or manner whatsoever, upon the penalty provided by the law to be duly and severely executed upon them." This was more than the Statute of Labourers prohibition on both begging and giving of alms. It had been a strictly economic gesture, an attempt to force people into the labour force. During the Black Death, the poor and infirm had been accepted as a natural element of the social order. Accepted, they were cared for, however inadequately. By the Stuart era a very negative view of the poor, especially vagrants and beggars, had developed. They were not a part of the natural order but rather a threat to it and to social stability.

The Lord Mayor's Orders even targeted dogs and cats, "capable of carrying the effluvia or infectious steams of bodies infected, even in their furs and hair." It was believed they could carry the plague from the infected to the well – and as a perceived disease vector they had to be exterminated. It is estimated that 40,000 dogs and 200,000 cats were slaughtered. Killing the latter would have been counterproductive as the rat population would have been freed of a predator. On the other hand, a related campaign to poison rats would have facilitated control of the disease.

Every attempt imaginable was made to break up the miasma. Cannons were fired and pots were banged. Resinous and sulphurous fires smouldered throughout the city. When an infected person died, the abode was fumigated. Parish workers, "burnt a great variety of fumes and perfumes in all the rooms, and made a great many smokes of pitch, of gunpowder, and of sulphur, all separately shifted; and washed their clothes, and the like." Public health measures, such as they were, aimed at clearing the miasma from the air.

Anxiety over infection, grief for dead family members, and social isolation in a sudden city of the dead all contributed to emerging signs of emotional strain. "It was seldom, that the weekly [mortality] bill came in, but there were two or three put in frighted, that is, that may well be called, frighted to death: But besides those, who were so frighted to die upon the spot, there were great numbers frighted to other extremes, some frighted out of their senses, some out of their memory, and some out of their understanding." While Defoe's narrator remains level-headed and dismisses most extraordinary rumours he is unable to resist one.

His suspension of disbelief is difficult to account for as he describes the physical impact of melancholia: "one in particular, who was so absolutely overcome with the pressure upon his spirits, that by degrees, his head sunk into his body, so between his shoulders, that the crown of his head was very little seen above the bones of his shoulders… the poor man never came to himself again, but anguished near a year in that condition and died: nor was he ever once seen to lift up his eyes, or to look upon any particular object." As absurd as this proposal is, one can only conclude that Defoe included the incident to demonstrate that even someone as level headed as his narrator was becoming increasingly credulous.

By August, Pepys's sense of foreboding is so strong he commits to updating his will, "Home, to draw over anew my will, which I had bound myself by oath to dispatch by tomorrow night; the town growing so unhealthy, that a man cannot depend upon living two days." Pepys even reports the pressure getting to the king: "Sept 7. Povy [Thomas Povy, MP for Bosiney, 1658 and Treasurer for Tangier] tells me by a letter he showed me, that the king is not, nor hath been of late, very well, but quite out of humour; and, as some think, in a consumption, and weary of every thing." A week later (Sept 14) Pepys himself seems to have an emotional crisis. Despite receiving word of a great naval victory by his mentor Lord Sandwich, he is overwhelmed by the plague's personal toll. His favourite watering hole, Angel's Tavern is shuttered and a list of dead acquaintances culminates with, "And, lastly, that both my servants, W. Hewer, and Tom Edwards, have lost their fathers, both in St Sepulchre's parish of the plague this week, do put me into great apprehension of melancholy, and with good reason."

While still blaming the air, not fleas, despite hundreds of years and dozens of visitations, the municipal government was getting it right for all the wrong reasons. Convinced that a miasma was the proximate cause of infection they quarantined the infected individuals, hoping to confine the miasma to the infected house, and banned social gatherings in enclosed spaces where the miasma of the infected might circulate. Those self-isolating were trying to keep the infected, but also the generalised miasmatic atmosphere, away from themselves and their kith and kin with them. The wealthy, fleeing the city, were escaping the miasmatic and sickening odour of the city, made the worse by the overwhelming number of corpses inadequately buried, if tended to at all.

In one comment, Defoe's narrator almost hit the nail on the head: "When all that will fly are gone, those that are left and must stand it, should stand stock still where they are, and not shift from one end of the town, or one part of the town to the other; for that is the bane and mischief of the whole, and they carry the plague from house to house in their very clothes." The fleas spreading the plague were, literally, being carried "in their very clothes." Isolation and social distancing were the only effective tools those remaining in London had.

On another occasion the narrator opines that if one is bitten by an infected person, one will also become infected: "Should one of those infected diseased creatures have bitten any man or woman, while the frenzy of the distemper was upon them, they, I mean the person so wounded, would as certainly have been incurably infected, as one that was sick before and had the tokens upon him." True for rabies, but not bubonic plague and more evidence of total ignorance of the plague's etiology.

Later, he offers another possibility, "I have heard, it was the opinion of others, that it might be distinguished by the party's breathing upon a piece of glass, where the breath condensing, there might living creatures be seen by a microscope of strange monstrous and frightful shapes, such as dragons, snakes, serpents, and devils, horrible to behold. But this I very much question the truth of, and we had no microscopes at that time, as I remember, to make the experiment with." Little did Defoe realise how right they were. Imagine, disease not divine punishment and miasmatic, but rather microbial.

Massive depopulation of the city of 460,000 pre-plague residents was the most direct and immediate impact of the plague. According to bills of mortality, between August 8 and October 10, 59,870 people died in London. Of those, fully 83%, slightly less than 50,000, were victims of the plague. The weekly toll peaked at over 7300 in late September. For the year the official tally was 68,590 killed by the plague, although Defoe's narrator puts it at "at least 100,000 of the plague only." Another contemporary, Lord Clarendon, estimated that the plague killed double the official figure. Thus, contemporary estimates ranged from one-third of the population to half of that.

Defoe's narrator takes note of increased unemployment and poverty as the epidemic progresses: "Certain it is, the greatest part of the poor, or families, who formerly lived by their labour, or by retail-trade, lived now on charity." He identifies five classes of activity negatively impacted. Manufacturers, from master workmen to apprentices; trade-related workers, from customs house clerks to carmen and porters; the building trades; the shipping trades, from sailors to rope and sail-makers; everyone involved in servicing and supplying the wealthy refugees from household staff left behind to book-keepers and barristers. Moreover, he adds, charity evaporated: "The distress of the poor was more now, a great deal than it was then, because all the sources of general charity were now shut: people supposed the main occasion to be over, and so stopped their hands; whereas particular objects were still very moving, and the distress of those that were poor, was very great indeed."

Defoe, himself a trader and investor, argues that employers attempted to mitigate the economic distress, "This stagnation of our manufacturing trade in the country, would have put the people there to much greater difficulties, but that the master-workmen, clothiers and others, to the uttermost of their stocks and strength kept on making their goods to keep the poor at work, believing that as soon as the sickness should abate they would have a quick demand in proportion to the decay of their trade at that time: but as none but those masters that were rich could do thus, and that many were poor and not able, the manufacturing trade in England suffered greatly, and the poor were pinched all over England by the calamity of the city of London only."

Pepys worries in October that the plague has hardened him, "Talking with him in the high way, come close by the bearers with a dead corpse of the plague; but, Lord! to see what custom is, that I am come almost to think nothing of it." Defoe, like chroniclers of the Black Death, regrets that the world seemed to be a more cankerous one after the plague. "With our infection, when it ceased, there did not cease the spirit of strife and contention, slander and reproach, which was really the great troubler of the nation's peace before… the quarrel remained, the church and the Presbyterians were incompatible." This quote introduces an important qualifier to the parish records. The [Anglican] Church only tracked Anglicans; Presbyterians, Quakers and Jews are never considered. As they were not baptised in the church there was no need to recognise their deaths. Inevitably, this implies that the parish records provide low figures in all instances.

Pepys's 'hardening' and Defoe's "spirit of strife and contention, slander and reproach" align with the survivors' chronicles of a meaner world in the wake of the Black Death. They also recall Frank Snowden's reference to "a mute despair... one might call post-traumatic stress." The two plagues are also similar in that they were both followed by significant depopulation and economic dislocation, the extent proportional to their scale. The Back Death pandemic killed one-third of Europe. The Great Plague of London killed one-third of a city.

The two, both products of *Yersinia pestis*, contrast in other ways. Most importantly, the two episodes demonstrate entirely different responses to plague. Nothing in the Black Death experience corresponds to the active efforts of the Lord Mayor and the city. Scientifically, nothing of significance had advanced. The disease was still wrongly believed to be airborne and a product of miasma. Nonetheless, it had also been learned that vigorous practical measures could constrain its spread and limit the human cost.

Those who could socially isolate through flight did – and that included the king and his court. In contrast, the Lord Mayor announced the City of London government was staying put. (Over and over again, pandemics bring out the best and worst in governments.) Those who could afford to hoard socially isolated that way. For the great unwashed, the Lord Mayor's orders were the best advice available. They strongly presage the situation in 2020. Bars and restaurants along with theatres and stadiums were closed to reduce community spread. The city became a ghost town and the economy shut down. Attempts were made at socially isolating the infected, with important contrasts to today. Then you were locked up as a default policy, infected until proven healthy. Today, people are told to socially isolate, which amounts to the same. The Lord Mayor even went so far as to publish lists of nostrums and concoctions thought to be effective. Helpfully, there were two – one for the poor and a more exotic one for the better off (Unicorn horn? Chloroquine? Bleach?). Unfortunately, while well intended, devoid of any scientific basis, they were often useless and occasionally dangerous.

The Lord Mayor's orders and attempts to lock up the infected met with considerable resistance from the populous. University of Vermont historian

Colby J Fischer found that, "the government operated under the false belief that the poor would agree that the safety of the London community out-weighed the well-being of a few individuals in quarantine." All of the strat-agems to avoid lockdown that Defoe laments were expressions of discontent with the Lord Mayor's orders and Colby concludes that this was unantici-pated, "The government and other members of the upper-class were shocked by the failure of the commoner to follow policy. Whether it was the urgent desire to meet with infected neighbours or the desire to attend funerals of friends and family, the failure to provide care for those in quarantine ensured its failure". The poor believed that they were being unfairly treated by the government, resulting in a resentment towards public health orders which hampered efforts to put them in place. These problems are not unfamiliar today to governments attempting to control the spread of COVID-19.

Inevitably, with the deaths, lockdowns and disruptions to trade there were short term economic consequences. in a striking parallel with modern times, it has also been suggested that the plague ruined many businesses – with erst-while customers remaining in their homes and concentrating what resources they had on the essentials such as food and fuel. Undercapitalised businesses and small tradespeople with the thinnest margins would have been culled from the marketplace. However, there are those too who believe that the longer term effects were less significant, with trade bouncing back and the English economy as a whole recovering rapidly.

The Black Death caused a decade long pause in the Hundred Years' War on the verge of English victory and saved the French monarch. It closed the door on Viking expansion in North America. In contrast, the Anglo-Dutch war took no notice of the Great Plague. The Dutch and the English contin-ued to batter one another in the Channel as the plague raged. On a purely quantitative level, passages about naval affairs are more frequent and more detailed than those on the plague in Pepys' diary. The plague, present in both countries, did not impact on the war's course or outcome.

Domestic politics were also little affected by the plague. Contemporaries and historians have since drawn a direct line from the Black Death through the Statute of Labourers to the Peasants' Revolt 30 years later. Less than 25 years after the London plague the Glorious Revolution (1688) occurred. However, no historian has ever suggested it was a consequence of the plague and it is accepted that it was another chapter in the royal Roman Catholic-Anglican disputes that had been ongoing since Henry VIII's reign.

The most notable outcome of the Great Plague of London is its lack of significant, long-term consequences. The economy, domestic politics and international affairs seem to have simply carried on business as usual. Possible factors accounting for this limited impact include its limited geographic extent – in the remainder of England there were only occasional outbreaks; its limited duration; and, the fact that only months after the plague abated the city was consumed by fire. The latter fact may explain why London never saw plague again. Building codes, possibly reflecting the city government's newfound influence, ordered that new construction use stone or brick rather than wood, which may have reduced the rat population. In contrast to these limited consequences, in the next chapter attention will turn to two infectious diseases that changed the fates of empires and emperors, and the course of history.

3.

Imperial Epidemics

"Take courage, I tell you, take courage.
The whites from France cannot hold out against us here in
Saint-Domingue.
They will fight well at first, but soon they will fall sick and die like flies."
Jean-Jacques Dessalines, First Emperor of Haiti

THE TERM Napoleon complex refers to men who are aggressive and quick to anger as compensation for being vertically challenged. The term is derived from Napoleon Bonaparte, the French general and emperor who is famous and was famously short. Except he wasn't. The metric system was only introduced in 1799 and not yet widely adopted, so the Emperor's height is commonly given in feet and inches, namely 5ft 2in. With the average male in the era standing 5ft 5in, the Emperor was short and so history has pronounced and popular opinion has confirmed. Except, the Emperor's height is in French units; converted to Imperial measure 5ft 2in in French units translates into almost 5ft 7in. The little squirt was actually slightly taller than average.

Conversely, his reputation as a military genius is rather larger than he deserves. He died in exile on a God-forsaken volcanic rock in the middle of the South Atlantic, when his final battle, Waterloo, ended in defeat. In the Americas his attempts to expand French influence and reassert French hegemony ended ignominiously. His expeditionary force was devastated, he lost sugar-rich Saint-Domingue (Haiti today) to revolution and was forced to sell Louisiana. In the east, his failed attempt to conquer Russia and his retreat from Moscow have become the textbook example of an army disintegrating. In the popular imagination, Napoleon's height has been shrunken and his reputation supersized. If failure is measured by the gap between ambitions and achievements, Napoleon comes up short – a three times loser.

Unremembered and unremarked is the role that pandemic disease played in his career's two most significant strategic setbacks. Napoleon's initiatives in the Caribbean were defeated more by *flavivirus* (the microbial causative agent of yellow fever) than rebellious slaves. The 65,000 troops and mariners he dispatched to Saint-Domingue jaundiced, bled from their eyes and ears, shivered as their temperature rose and died of yellow fever. The plan to subdue the island and use it as a launching pad for an invasion of North America through Louisiana and up the Mississippi valley evaporated.

A decade later, on the eastern edge of his European Empire, Napoleon launched the Grande Armée's pan-European forces against Russia. From the Pripet Marshes north to the Baltic Sea, more than half a million men and camp followers, and half again the number of horses, surged toward Moscow in June 1812. Within weeks they were dying of dysentery. Inconclusively earning a marginal victory in early September at Borodino, they struggled on to Moscow. Unable to feed and shelter themselves over the impending winter, as their numbers steadily declined, in mid-October they turned southwest and began to march home. Typhus broke out, the retreat descended into a rout and men froze to death where they fell. Dysentery killed at least 150,000 during the trek to Moscow and typhus killed half the survivors during the chaotic flight. Nine out of ten members of the Grande Armée died, with fewer than 70,000 making it back across the River Niemen. It is said that Russia is often best defended by Generals Mud and Winter, but in 1812 it was Generals Rickettsia and Shigella (the bacterial sources of typhus and dysentery) that saved the day. Twice pandemics left the Emperor's strategic plans in tatters and transformed the map, and the very history, of the globe from India to the Continental Divide in western North America.

Hispaniola is the second largest island in the Greater Antilles archipelago, due east of Cuba. It was Columbus' first landfall in the Americas and the following year, in 1493, he introduced sugarcane to the island. The Treaty of Ryswick in 1697 required Spain to cede the western third of the island to France. It quickly became the most valuable colony in the West Indies, earning the nickname, 'Pearl of the Antilles'. A plantation system predicated on slave labour produced vast quantities of sugar and coffee. It also served as a logistical hub for French possessions in the Caribbean and North America, particularly France's vast holdings north and west of the mouth of the Mississippi River known as the Louisiana Territory.

Throughout the Antilles, the Caribbean and the southern portion of French Louisiana yellow fever is still endemic today, with occasional epidemic episodes. (In New Orleans in 1853 it would kill almost 8000 in a city of 115,000 and in 1796 it had already killed 700 in a city of 8,500.) Yellow fever is an RNA virus. The CDC summarises its etiology: "Yellow fever virus is transmitted to people primarily through the bite of infected *Aedes* or *Haemagogus* species mosquitoes. Mosquitoes acquire the virus by feeding on infected primates (human or non-human) and then can transmit the virus to other primates (human or non-human)." Infected individuals are asymptomatic for three to six days, then patients exhibit sudden onset of fever, chills and severe headache. In Saint-Domingue it was endemic at a rate of about 3% annually. Facing harsh daily work and horrible living conditions, slaves were estimated to have a life cycle of only five years. As many as 40,000 had to be imported annually to replace losses. Even 200 years ago the bountiful Pearl of the Antilles had a depraved downside.

When Napoleon assumed control of French foreign affairs they had, in the Americas, been in decline for 50 years. In 1750, France controlled North America's destiny, yet by the turn of the century they were reduced to bit part players, on the verge of losing any role. At mid-century they had the colony New France along the St Lawrence River and northwest into the fur trade country. They also laid claim to the gigantic Louisiana Territory, the middle of the continent from the Mississippi to the mountains, 828,000 square miles, fully one-quarter of the continental USA today . The two claims theoretically met around the Montana-Saskatchewan border creating an arc of French territory up the Mississippi and west from New France that confined the British colonies to the Atlantic coast.

Fifty years later the balance of power had swung decisively against the French. On September 13, 1759, the British captured the cliff top fortress of Quebec City. At the ensuing Treaty of Paris in 1763 France lost all of its possessions in northern North America with the exception of two small islands. The dual French pincers enveloping the coastal colonies had lost a wing. In the future the two players in the region would be the British and the former colonies that became the United States of America, both competitively racing westward. Subsequently, a slave revolt in Saint-Domingue disrupted the flow of lucre from the colony and threatened its key role as a transportation and supply hub amid the remaining French possessions in the Caribbean. In North America, when Napoleon assumed power, France's northern power base was no more and its position in the south was tenuous.

Born Napulione Buonaparte on the island of Corsica, son of a minor Italian noble, educated at a military academy in northern France and then the École Militaire in Paris, he trained as an artillery officer. In October 1795 he assumed authority over his nominal superior Paul Barras, suppressed a Royalist revolt in Paris and wooed Barras' mistress, Joséphine de Beauharnais. A grateful revolutionary government made him commander of the French Army in Italy. He married Joséphine, departed for Italy and within a year had defeated the Austrians and installed compliant sister republics across northern Italy. In 1798 he began campaigning in the eastern Mediterranean and Egypt. A see-saw campaign marked by victories on land and defeats at sea followed.

His troops did not blast the nose off the Sphinx. They couldn't have; sketches from 50 years earlier show the Sphinx already a victim of a rhinotomy. Indeed, his troops were accompanied by a smaller army of scholars. While engineers and geodesists were there to plan what would become the Suez Canal, there were also Orientalists, naturalists and historians. Among their equipment was a printing press with French, Arabic and Greek sets of typeface. Their initial enthusiastic efforts at archaeology often wrought damage due to inexperience, but belligerently obliterating antiquities was not on their enlightenment agenda.

Meanwhile, in France military defeats and popular discontent again threatened the governing Directorate. Secretly, Napoleon abandoned his army (for the first time) and returned to Paris. This time he proved no saviour of the government. On 18th Brumaire in the revolutionary calendar (November 9, 1799), he led a coup d'état that established the Consulate. Napoleon was appointed First Consul for a decade and given the authority to appoint the other two consuls who had only advisory power. Bonaparte was on his way to becoming emperor. No longer a mere artillery officer, he was in charge of grand strategy.

His attention turned to the Americas. He wanted the vast and largely unexplored Louisiana territory occupied and developed to prevent western expansion of the newborn American Republic and British North America. However, first the problem of a rebellious and increasingly autonomous Saint-Domingue had to be settled. The island produced more sugar, 'white gold', than all of Great Britain's Caribbean possessions combined. It required 1600 ships a year to get the commodity to France.

However, in August 1791, led by François-Dominique Toussaint Louverture, the slaves in Saint-Domingue rose up in a massive revolt, killing thousands of French planters but suffering casualties themselves in reprisals. For a dozen years the Assembly in Paris debated what to do while the planters and *maroons* – escaped slaves living freely in the hills and forests – fought a vicious guerilla war with frequent atrocities committed by both sides.

By the time Napoleon took power the situation was incredibly complicated. The revolutionary French assembly had abolished slavery, but the planters on the island refused to accept that. Both the British and Spanish had tried to intervene and retreated chastened. To Napoleon issues of slavery, legality and ethics were all incidental: he sided with the planters, not the Republic. Geopolitics demanded that the colony be pacified and stable before it could provide a secure base for expansion into the heart of North America. In a letter to his Minister of Marine, Napoleon made his ultimate objective clear: "My intention, Citizen Minister, is that we take possession of Louisiana with the shortest possible delay, that this expedition be organised in the greatest secrecy, and that it have the appearance of being directed on St Domingo. The troops that I intend for it being on the Scheldt, I should like them to depart from Antwerp or Flushing." Napoleon prepared two expeditionary forces. The first to restore French authority in Saint-Domingue, the second to invade Louisiana. This latter fleet was assembled but never sailed due to events in Saint-Domingue.

Napoleon dispatched General Victor Emmanuel Charles Leclerc, commanding a force eventually reinforced to over 60,000 soldiers and sailors, to Saint-Domingue. It was a force even larger than he, Napoleon, had taken to Egypt. Leclerc was married to Napoleon's famously beautiful and infamously amorous little sister, Pauline. It has been suggested he was chosen to command the expedition not as a sign of competence or Imperial favour, but as a nod to Pauline. She wanted him out of her way, and the move worked in a big way when 'yellow jack' killed him before the year was out.

The French arrived at Saint-Domingue on February 2, 1802. They landed on the north shore of the island near the port of Le Cap. The plan was to fight their way into Le Cap and establish a firm base of operations in a resupply port. Subsequently, five independent columns would traverse the colony forcing the enemy into a decisive battle where they would be destroyed.

Louverture had different ideas. His forces fled for the safety of the interior wilderness, leaving Le Cap to the French. The French entered a heap of smouldering ruins and a destroyed port. The rebels totally immolated the town. The 'victorious' French captured no supplies, had no shelter and held the deed to a largely useless port.

After two weeks, Leclerc launched his search and destroy mission. Supremely confident that a European army could not be defeated by disorganised rebels, and deeming maps unnecessary, they headed into the heart of darkness on Wednesday, February 17. Things went south quickly. The soldiers sweated and stumbled in heavy wool uniforms and shoddy boots. Blindly plunging forward, they were harassed by ambushes and hit and run attacks by an enemy who knew the terrain intimately and had an extensive intelligence network. The French could not move without Louverture being informed, while they never knew where or when the *maroons* would strike. The French sought a decisive battle but the rebels refused to provide it. Instead the French endured daily attrition, exhaustion and frustration. There followed three months of savage irregular warfare, with the French becoming increasingly violent in their reprisals.

Despite the defection to the French of rebel leader Henri Christophe and the capture of Toussaint Louverture in April, the guerrilla warfare continued. It carried on into the rainy, summer season, the mosquito population blew up with the rain, and the French began to sicken and die. Leclerc could only lament his troops' infirmity: "You will see that the army which you calculated at 26,000 men is reduced at this moment to 12,000. At this moment I have 3600 men in the hospital. In the last fortnight I have lost 30-50 men a day in the colony, and there is no day when 200-250 men do not enter the hospital, while no more than 50 come out." Fittingly in the context of voodoo-influenced Saint-Domingue, on what is now Haiti, General Leclerc was himself felled by 'yellow jack' on November 2, the Day of the Dead.

The disease had a case fatality rate approaching 50% among Leclerc's forces. That is exponentially higher than the endemic rate of approximately 3% on Saint-Domingue. It also greatly exceeds the CFR for other yellow fever epidemics in the Americas. In terms of mortality, Leclerc's approximately 40,000 fatal casualties and a total death toll in the colony of 55,000 far exceeds the butcher's bill for the 1878 Mississippi River valley epidemic that killed 20,000 or the 5000 that paid the price in Philadelphia in 1793 and again 80 years later. The epidemic among the French expeditionary force to Saint-Domingue was the largest yellow fever epidemic in history, with the highest case fatality rate ever recorded. It affected a specific demographic (the French expeditionary force), in a specific locale (Saint-Domingue) for a limited period of time (six months). On the other hand, its infectiousness and virulence, its savagery and its global implications all point to its significance.

The extreme severity of the epidemic, as is frequently the case, was the confluence of a perfect storm of circumstances for both the microbe, *flavivirus*, the vector, *Aedes aegypti* (the Egyptian mosquito) and the virgin population host. Earlier, the Black Death was referred to as a 'virgin soil' pandemic; the bacteria was moving into new territory. In that paradigm the 1802 yellow fever epidemic in Saint-Domingue was a 'virgin population' epidemic. The virus did not spread to new victims but rather a virgin population, the expeditionary force, came to it. The French troops had no immunity to yellow fever. They were immunologically naive hosts.

And they were leaping into a vast reservoir of infected individuals. Yellow fever was endemic in Saint-Domingue. The importation of tens of thousands of slaves annually and the regular comings and goings of European sailors, merchants and bureaucrats provided the virus with candidates for infection and ensured the disease remained endemic. Conversely, many slaves were already immune when they arrived from Africa where yellow fever was also endemic. Others were infected on the island and had recovered and were immune before the expeditionary force arrived. Consequently, Louverture's force had high levels of immunity: Their opponents were virgins.

The timing of operations also favoured the virus. The destruction of Le Cap delayed the French and pushed operations into the rainy mosquito breeding season, from April to June, and the troops were forced to slog through clouds of disease-carrying blood-suckers while up to their knees in water and mud in the jungle.

What is truly remarkable is that the rebel leaders knew what they were doing. They realised that they were buying time until microbial reinforcements arrived and if they could simply hold out that long, yellow fever would do their work for them. In a letter to his subordinate General Jean-Jacques Dessalines, Louverture wrote, we have to wait "for the rainy season, which will rid us of our enemies…" All they had to do was stall and victory would eventually be theirs.

As he prepared his troops for their first confrontation with the French in March 1802, Louverture's successor as commander, Dessalines, told them, "Take courage, I tell you, take courage. The whites from France cannot hold out against us here in Saint-Domingue. They will fight well at first, but soon they will fall sick and die like flies." The Haitian Declaration of Independence even gives a nod to the disease in its dismissal of all things French Republic, "The difference between its cruelty and our patient moderation, its color and ours, the great seas that separate us, our avenging climate, all tell us plainly that they are not our brothers, that they never will be, and that if they find refuge among us, they will plot again to trouble and divide us."

The disease was being treated as a reliable military tactic. The claim that the Khan catapulted infected cadavers into Kaffa with the intent to spread disease is questionable at best. That being the case, the Haitian War of Independence is the first clear and documented example of microbes deployed as a weapon system – with Louverture and Dessalines fully aware of what they were doing. The Haitian rebels weaponised yellow fever during the struggle against Napoleon.

Rebellious slaves, non-Europeans, allied with *flavivirus* had defeated a disciplined European army and, indeed, the Emperor himself. And their success had global consequences. It changed the rules of the game. For the first time, according to Johns Hopkins University historian Franklin W. Knight, slaves "overthrew both their colonial status and its economic system and established a new political state of entirely free individuals – with some ex-slaves constituting the new political authority." It established the fact that non-European slaves could defeat and oust their masters politically and economically.

The global shockwaves that followed changed the map of North America and the course of its history. They doubled the size of the United States and set the stage for its rapid economic and demographic expansion as well as its geographic drive westward. Arguably this made conflict between indigenous nations resident in the Territory and the United States inevitable, leading to decades of often genocidal conflicts (occasionally accompanied by epidemics) at tragic cost. French control of the Louisiana Territory would have precluded the USA from growing to extend from coast to coast. An isolated epidemic with 50,000 fatalities changed the course of North American history substantially and forever.

Fifty years later, during the American Civil War, a second attempt was made to employ yellow fever as a biological weapon. Dr Luke Blackwood was a Kentucky backwoods charlatan with a reputation as a yellow fever specialist. He was also a rabid Confederate. Together with Haligonian Alexander Keith (not the famous brewer but rather his psychopathic nephew), he planned to kill President Lincoln and infect the Union with yellow fever in 1863. Blackburn would ship soiled bedding and clothing from yellow fever patients in Bermuda to Keith, who would forward them to destinations across the north. The conspirators planned to send an especially fine suit and shirts exposed to yellow fever to President Abraham Lincoln himself. The delivery man, Geoffrey Hyams, lost his nerve however – foiling that part of the plot. The entire scheme was pointless because the lynchpin, the mosquito, was not in on the play. Yellow fever victims' bedding is not infectious; the only vector is the mosquito. Ironically, the Haitians employed biological warfare passively, they just let it happen, and it succeeded while Blackburn and Keith actively attempted to weaponise it and failed.

Spanked in North America, Napoleon's situation was no better in Europe. Three months after Haiti (its original Arawak name) proclaimed independence on New Year's Day 1803, England declared war on France. Over the next two years they imposed a blockade on Europe and destroyed any French naval plans at the battles of Finnisterre and Trafalger. An agreement with Sweden followed and then the Tsar provided the backbone of the Third Coalition, impressing the Austrian and Holy Roman Emperors enough that they signed on.

It was a mistake. With a series of brilliant manoeuvres combining mobility with firepower, Napoleon bested the Coalition. His tactics at the battle of Ulm in September 1805 are still taught in military academies and known simply as the 'Ulm manoeuvre'. A month later he captured Vienna and at Austerlitz he smashed the combined forces of Russia and Austria in what many regard as the Grande Armée's greatest victory. The Emperor concurred. "The battle of Austerlitz is the finest of all I have fought", he once exulted.

In 1807 the Treaties of Tilsit imposed heavy indemnities and other humiliating conditions on Austria and Russia. The year before Napoleon had reorganised the former Holy Roman Empire into the Confederation of the Rhine. In May 1812, the Emperor assembled his minions in Dresden along with Francis II, Emperor of Austria. After watching an intimidating march past by the Grande Armée, the Emperor solicited donations of troops for his pending invasion of Russia.

As a result, when the Grande Armée crossed the Nieman it was a polyglot force. The largest allied contingent was 90,000 Poles hoping Napoleon's victory would lead to gains for their vassal state, the Duchy of Warsaw, at the expense of Russia. Half that number of troops came from the northern Italian kingdoms the Emperor had established a decade earlier. The members of the Confederation of the Rhine all provided tiny contingents. As a result estimates of Napoleon's strength cover a wide range, from 500,000 to almost one million. Regardless of the precise figures, it was the largest military force ever assembled to that time in human history, ten times the size of the Saint-Domingue expeditionary force.

Historians have long debated Napoleon's motives. Ending serfdom and respect for Polish national unification do not even merit consideration, although they were the public excuses. A more plausible thesis is that the Tsar was still too close to the English, particularly in a mercantile sense, and undermining Napoleon's Continental System by violating the embargo on trade with England.

The best evidence is Napoleon's own words. Louis Marie Jacques Amalric, comte de Narbonne-Lara was Napoleon's most trusted diplomatic advisor, the equivalent of a Foreign Minister or Secretary of State. When Napoleon wanted to ascertain King William III of Prussia's response to a possible invasion of Russia he dispatched Narbonne-Lara to Potsdam. He also delivered the ultimatum to Tsar Alexander I in Vilnus. There is every reason to believe that Napoleon shared with him his innermost thoughts. Russia was merely a waystation on the road to India, "Now we shall march on Moscow, and from Moscow why not turn to India." Frustrated by British intransigence and continuing belligerence, the Grande Armée would wheel south after wintering in Moscow and conquer the Raj, 'Let no one tell Napoleon that it is far from Moscow to India. Alexander of Macedon had to travel a long way from Greece to India, but did that stop him? Alexander reached the Ganges, having started from a point as distant as Moscow." He concluded, "Then tell me, will it be so impossible for the French army to reach the Ganges? And once the French sword touches the Ganges, the edifice of England's mercantile greatness will tumble in ruins." His plans to invade England had been repeatedly frustrated so he proposed to attack the jewel in the crown by land, across the Caucasus and through Afghanistan.

In terms of Napoleon's strategic thinking there is more to this proposal than first meets the eye. Recall that Saint-Domingue was not a final objective, just a base of operations for French exploitation of the Louisiana Territory. Similarly, Russia was to provide a secure base for an indirect strike at English economic power. Regardless, in both instances the preliminaries were defeated by epidemics and grand strategy rendered moot.

It took three days, using three bridges, for the Grande Armée, its 250,000 horses and 50,000 camp followers to cross the Nieman. Napoleon planned to strike the boundary between the two Russian armies facing him, split them apart and, in succession, destroy each in detail. Then the Tsar would sue for peace and the campaign would end without the inconvenience of a trek to Moscow. The Russians refused to comply, slowly retreating instead and refusing to confront the Grande Armée.

As the advance continued, the Grande Armée began to fall apart at the seams due to its size. A huge army required an equivalently huge number of uniforms and boots. Napoleon bought the cheapest machine-made uniforms and boots with glued rather than stitched soles. By the battle of Borodino in September, many of the French infantry were unshod. Napoleon's style of combat – phenomenal mobility – was also proving untenable in Russia. Speed had its price. Napoleon's soldiers were expected to plunder, otherwise they would have starved and frozen. They carried nothing beyond their weapons and tools. No blankets, no rations, no tents and a minimal baggage train with no forges or bakers' ovens and neither medication nor medical supplies.

In heavily populated and developed western Europe, this was a brilliant approach. If the French needed lumber or flour they simply took it, or took over the entire mill. Similarly, blacksmiths worked in shops they could take at gunpoint. Tents were redundant because civilian housing could be obtained by simply throwing out the occupants. According to General Philippe de Ségur, there was also a psychological benefit, "Napoleon was well aware of the attraction which that mode of subsistence had for the soldier; that it made him love war, because it enriched him; that it gratified him, by the authority which it frequently gave him over classes superior to his own; that in his eyes it had all the charms of a war of the poor against the rich." But the Grande Armée was a behemoth, the equivalent of the population of the city of Paris moving across the landscape. The system of plunder had never been tried on this large a scale.

In European Russia the system was doomed before a shot was fired. In 1812 it was largely a trackless wilderness with only a handful of significant towns connected by a primitive road network. There was no civilian housing to be requisitioned. There were few mills to grind flour for bread. (Without a mill, grain is good for nothing but distilling and distilleries were also few and far between.) The system of plunder was impossible because there was nothing to plunder.

The Russians knew this, or at least their brilliant German military advisors did. Smolensk is closer to Moscow than the Nieman by 500 miles and General Gerhard von Scharnhost insisted that battle must be avoided for those first 500 miles of the French advance. Military theorist Carl von Clausewitz agreed: "Bonaparte must totally fail, by virtue of the great dimensions of the Russian empire, if these should only be brought sufficiently into play… an idea that could not fail to be beneficial if carried out to the extent of not shrinking from evacuating the whole country as far as Smolensk, and only beginning the war in earnest from that point." In fact, the first decisive shot was not fired until Borodino, a mere 70 miles from Moscow.

Unbeknownst to the Grande Armée, a Fifth Column was beginning to operate within their ranks. Schigellosis. Widely known as dysentery, it is a result of infection with *Schigella* bacteria. Transmission is oral-fecal: the sufferer becomes infected by ingesting food or water tainted with fecal matter and then begins infecting others by shedding the virus in their stool. And dysentery is incredibly virulent – a very small bacterial load is able to overwhelm the immune system. The bacteria attack the epithelial cells in the colon, producing a toxin. Death can occur within hours, but five to seven days is typical.

In 1823, Scottish physician Sir George Ballingall, regius professor of military surgery at the University of Edinburgh, described the vile symptoms of the disease in *Practical Observations on Fever, Dysentery, and Liver Complaints*. Initially fever, rapid pulse and abdominal pain. Then malodorous diarrhea that is "discharged with more or less explosive force... [and] exactly resembles water in which raw flesh has been macerated." Symptoms of dehydration develop including cold sweat, furred tongue, sunken eyes and nausea. Any fluids given are immediately vomited. Stupor, coma and death follow inevitably.

A schigellosis infection confers no immunity. Thus, each member of the Grande Armée was a candidate. More importantly, in Frank Snowden's memorable turn of phrase, the Grande Armée was operating "in a microenvironment of their own creation that rivalled the appalling sanitary conditions of a dense urban slum." Napoleon's soldiers were not living in a pigsty, they were living in a cesspit. Issues surrounding urbanisation, sanitation and oral-fecal transmission are central to 19th century pandemics as the following chapter on cholera will also demonstrate.

On the march, the Grande Armée's columns stretched over 20 miles. More than a day's march and everyone suffered for this except the vanguard. They marched on roads and across fields turned to a gelatinous mush, liberally mixed with horse manure. Lacking shelter, they bedded down in it also. Any firewood would have been consumed by the head of the column, as was food. Safe drinking water was impossible to obtain and in the context of dysentery that meant the R-nought number was astronomical. Troops cooked with and drank water that those ahead of them had washed their diarrhea-soaked drawers in. Food cooked communally and distributed with filthy hands spread bacteria. Accompanying Napoleon's troops would have been a massive, sky darkening cloud of buzzing flies. And every fly had the potential to spread *schigella* on its hairy legs and as it regurgitated before each meal. With no medication or supplies, the Grande Armée's medical services were helpless, reduced to scouring the fields and woods for medicinal herbs. Infection raced through the ranks.

The fluidity of the situation and the impending holocaust make statistical sources rare and calculations difficult. Imprecise medical terminology also makes it difficult to differentiate between dysentery and multiple other gastrointestinal ailments that chronically infected soldiers. A widely mooted figure is 4000 deaths per day by August, prior to the decisive engagement of the campaign. A week after Borodino, on September 14, the Grande Armée entered Moscow, at least the two-thirds still alive did. Approximately 200,000 soldiers had died of disease and malnutrition or deserted. In contrast, at Borodino, the largest single battle of the Napoleonic Wars, the French suffered 30,000 fatalities. For every French soldier killed by the enemy, seven died of disease, primarily the dysentery epidemic.

Finally, Moscow would offer relief from their filthy, nomadic life and secure winter quarters. Taking a page out of the Louverture playbook, Russian commander General Mikhail Kutuzov, evacuated the city and set up defensive positions to the east. Unknown to the French, all of the city's firefighting equipment had been destroyed. The next day as Russian arsonists ignited stores of blackpowder, the French were forced to watch the city burn to the ground around them. When Napoleon occupied Vienna in the fall of 1805 it was intact and well stocked, it also offered up 100,000 muskets and 500 cannon. Moscow offered nothing.

After a month of lingering, looting and indecision, the Emperor finally accepted reality, encouraged by a blizzard on October 15. The Grande Armée was no longer a predator. When it fled Moscow it had become prey. Long forgotten is an apparently minor battle of immense epidemiological importance. The town of Malo-Jaroslavetz, on the Luzha River lies 40 miles southwest of Moscow. It is the point at which the road west splits into northern and southern routes. The French had marched to Moscow on the northern branch and intended to flee on the unspoiled and unsoiled southern route. At Malo-Jaroslavetz, General Dmitry Sergeyevich Dokhturov's infantry blocking force nudged Napoleon's vanguard, the IV Italian Corps commanded by the Emperor's son-in-law, Eugène Rose de Beauharnais, Duke of Leuchtenberg north. The Grande Armée was forced to retrace its route on the northern branch. On the way in they had polluted the water and wells, denuded the land of food and firewood and consumed all the livestock: This empty, slimy, polluted land was home to what was fast becoming a mob for the next seven weeks as they tramped west.

Fate was not yet done with the increasingly desperate rabble though. Typhus struck. Typhus does not involve oral-fecal transmission and, while totally unrelated, it shares a similar vector to bubonic plague, relying on the human louse. Uniquely, however it relies on both the oral and fecal aspects of the louse. A louse defecates as it feeds and like a mosquito the salivary lubricant facilitating the bite is irritating. When the human victim scratches the bite they introduce the loose louse fecal matter into the bloodstream.

Bitten by an infected louse, scratching introducing the bacteria into the bloodstream, it multiplies within the cells of the major organs – the brain, lungs, kidneys, liver and heart. The pace of reproduction is violently rapid and the individual cells begin exploding, causing massive internal blood loss and agonising pain. Dyskinetic jerks accompany delirium and hallucinations. It is both a gruesome death to suffer and a terrifying sight to witness. One made all the more likely by the increasing malnourishment of its starving hosts. Every day the weather grew colder. While this suppressed dysentery, it facilitated typhus as freezing men pulled clothing off the dying and slept together in heaps to stay warm at night.

Even worse, according to multiple memoirs, was the ceaseless, agonising irritation of a body swarming with biting lice. In his memoirs, Sergeant Adrien Jean Baptiste François Bourgogne wrote, "I had slept for an hour when I felt an unbearable tingling over the whole of my body... and to my horror discovered that I was covered with vermin! I jumped up, and in less than two minutes was as naked as a new-born babe, having thrown my shirt and trousers into the fire. The crackling they made was like a brisk firing..."

Starvation brought on theft and murder. Raymond A. P. J. de Fezensac, Aide-de-Camp to Louis-Ferdinand Berthier, Chief of Staff to Napoleon remembered, "Our soldiers, famishing, hesitated not to seize by force the provisions of every isolated man they came across, and the latter considered themselves lucky if their clothes were not also torn from their backs. After having ravaged the whole country, we were thus reduced to destroying ourselves." Eventually, cannibalism began occurring. It is fascinating to read the verbal gymnastics of Sergeant Bourgogne as he explains how it was only sensible to eat human flesh although he personally, of course, never indulged. "I am sure that if I had not found any horseflesh myself, I could have turned cannibal. To understand the situation, one must have felt the madness of hunger; failing a man to eat, one could have demolished the devil himself, if he were only cooked."

In early November, the Russians entered Dorogobuzh, 35 miles east of Smolensk in the wake of the fleeing French. General Robert Wilson, the British military commissioner, accompanied them and saw gruesome evidence of an impoverished, ill-clad, undisciplined mob: "The naked masses of dead and dying men; the mangled carcasses of 10,000 horses, which had, in some cases, been cut for food before life had ceased, the craving of famine at other points forming groups of cannibals; the air enveloped in flame and smoke; the prayers of hundreds of naked wretches, flying from the peasantry whose shouts of vengeance echoed incessantly through the woods… formed such a scene as probably was never witnessed to such an extent in the history of the world."

A month later when they encountered Napoleon's abandoned wounded in Vilṇa, Lithuania, the situation was even worse. That day, December 9, the emperor, disguised as a common soldier, abandoned his army and fled for Paris. Smoke and stink from dung fires in the streets intended to break up the miasma lingered. December in Lithuania meant the weather was frigid and every last stick of firewood, every flammable item, had been vacuumed up by the fleeing mob that had once been the Grande Armée. "The hospital at St Bazile presented the most awful and hideous sight: 7500 bodies were piled like pigs of lead over one another in the corridors... and all the broken windows and walls were stuffed with feet, legs, arms, hands, trunks and heads to fit the apertures, and keep out the air from the yet living," Wilson noted.

Five months after swarming over the Nieman in June, the dazed survivors of the Grande Armée, freezing and starving, returned. They had suffered an unheard of 90% casualty rate, and the vast majority died of infectious diseases, first dysentery and then typhus. There were a host of other contributing factors from sheer distance to hubris, from the failure to commit the Imperial Guard at Borodino to the decision to tarry in the smouldering ruins of Moscow, but it was consecutive epidemics – not defeat on the field of battle nor even the cold and starvation – that annihilated the Grande Armée.

On two continents, three epidemic diseases had ravaged French forces. Military historians can debate endlessly issues of strategy and tactics but it is epidemiologists that hold the key to Napoleon's defeats at both edges of his empire. Yellow fever, not combat, destroyed Napoleon's Saint Domingue expeditionary force. Yellow fever brought to power, for the first time, a revolutionary government that had overthrown both the slave economy and their colonial political masters. An epidemic that had a mere, by pandemic standards, 50,000 fatalities changed the course of North American history.

In Russia, Napoleon's army, the largest military force in the world, was wiped out not at Borodino, but by dysentery and typhus. The loss of veterans meant the emperor's armies were never as well trained or experienced again. Mosquitoes, lice and bad water destroyed his grand imperial ambitions.

There is also an interesting epilogue to this story concerning French civil engineer Charles Joseph Minard. Born in Dijon in 1781 and educated at the École nationale des ponts et chaussées in Paris, he worked on major civil engineering projects across Europe throughout his career. However, his passion was thematic mapping and his graphic representation of the Grande Armée is regarded as one of the finest, and probably the first, examples of flow mapping. The X-axis represents the distance from the Nieman River to Moscow, and is augmented by a temperature line below. The map depicts the Grande Armée as an irregular brown arrow advancing to, and black arrow retreating from, Moscow. The width of the arrow indicates the number of troops. The Grand Armée is initially a thick brown base that steadily shrinks as it moves east. Retreating from Moscow a narrow black arrow diminishes to a trickle. It was produced in 1869, an era considered the golden age of cartography. It is a fitting introduction to 'King Cholera' as epidemiological mapping plays a central role in its story also.

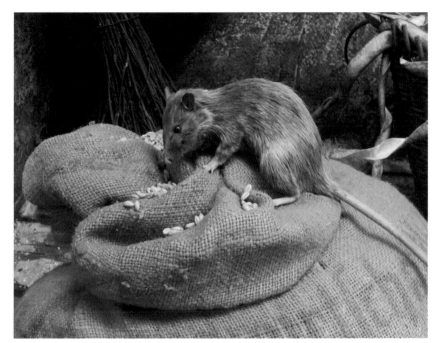

This pesky little critter, *Rattus rattus*, carried the *Xenopsylla cheopis* (Oriental rat flea) that carried *Yersinia pestis* (bubonic plague bacteria) into Europe in 1347.

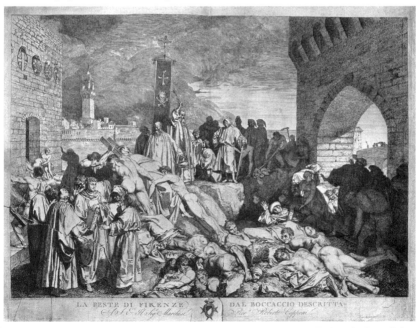

LA PESTE DI FIRENZE   DAL BOCCACCIO DESCRITTA

The plague of Florence in 1348, as described in Boccaccio's *The Decameron*. Etching by Luigi Sabatelli the Elder (1772-1850).

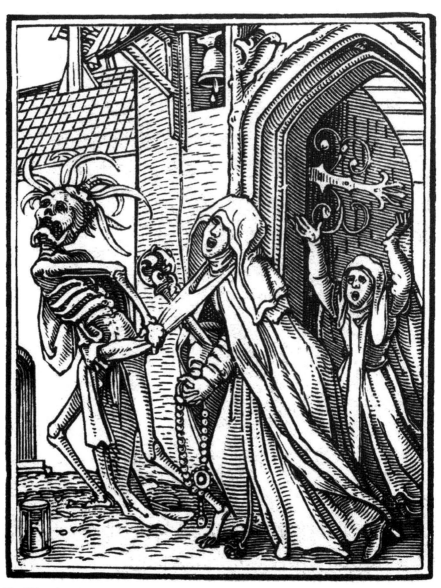

The Abbess from Hans Holbein's *Simolachri, Historie, e Figure de la Morte*, 1549. Despite her religiosity and her rosary even the Abbess must come when death calls.

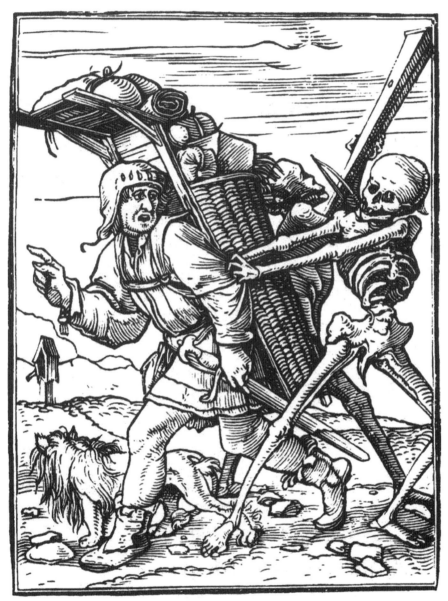

The Pedlar from Hans Holbein's *Simolachri, Historie, e Figure de la Morte*, 1549. Pointing to his destination and loaded with goods the pedlar cannot hurry away when death tugs at his sleeve.

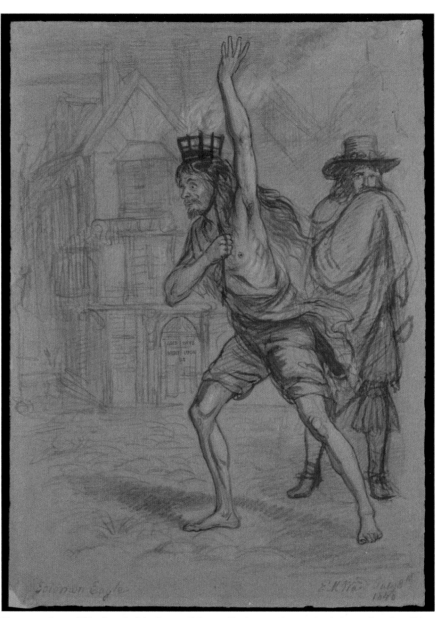

"I suppose the world has heard of the famous Solomon Eagle an enthusiast: he tho' not infected at all, but in his head; went about denouncing of judgement upon the city in a frightful manner; sometimes quite naked, and with a pan of burning charcoal on his head." –Daniel Defoe

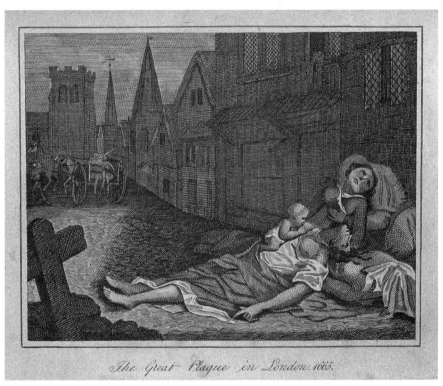

The Great Plague in London. 1665.

Two women lying dead in a London street during the great plague, 1665, one with a child who is still alive. Etching after R. Pollard II.

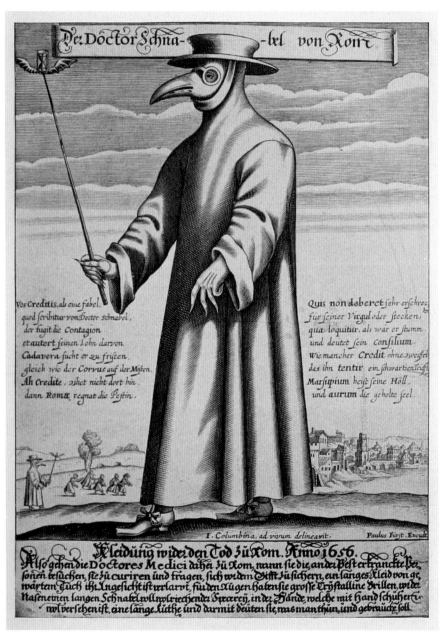

Paul Fürst, engraving, c. 1721, of a plague doctor of Marseilles (introduced as 'Dr Beaky of Rome'). His nose-case is filled with herbal material to keep off the plague.

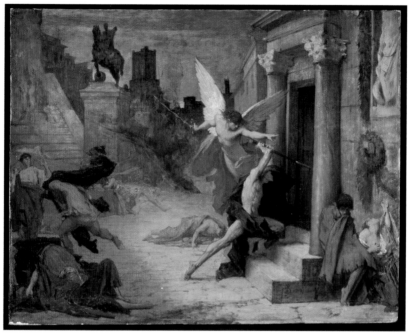

The artist of this painting took inspiration from a passage in Jacobus de Voragine's 13th-century 'Golden Legend', which describes how divine vengeance brought a plague to Rome. In the painting, plague-stricken figures lie in torment in the streets, while to the right, a good angel commands the bad angel to strike with his spear the homes where the plague will enter.

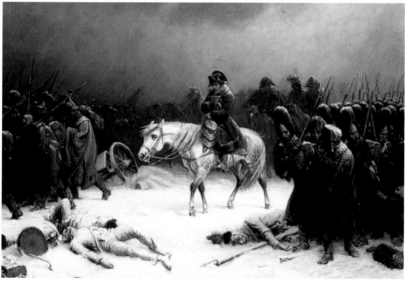

Decimated by dysentery and typhus, ill clad and underfed, the remains of the Grande Armée retreat from Moscow. Pandemic typhus and dysentery killed far more of Napoleon's soldiers than the enemy.

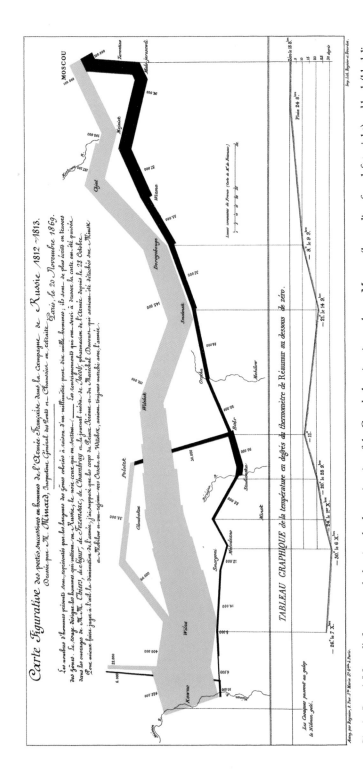

Charles Joseph Minard's famous graph showing the decreasing size of the Grande Armée as it marches to Moscow (brown line, from left to right) and back (black line, from right to left) with the size of the army equal to the width of the line. Temperature is plotted on the lower graph for the return journey (multiply Réaumur temperatures by 1¼ to get Celsius, e.g. −30°R = −37.5°C).

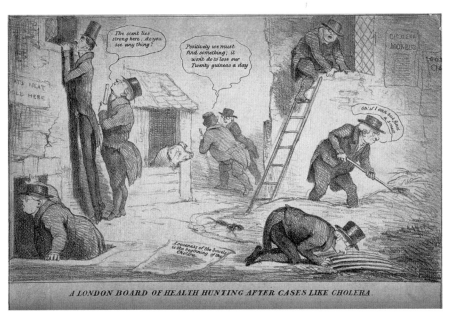

Amused, a sow looks on as the London Board of Health search for signs of cholera, 'Positively we must find something; it wont do to lose our twenty guineas a day.' Other than in the midst of a pandemic public health officials have always been accused of wasting money on needless preparation.

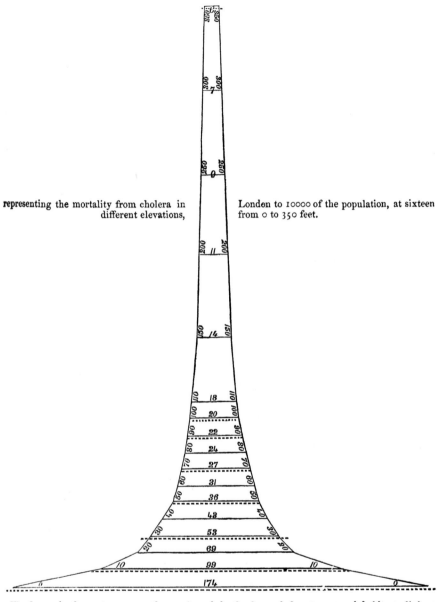

representing the mortality from cholera in different elevations,

London to 10000 of the population, at sixteen from 0 to 350 feet.

The figures in the centre express the number of deaths from cholera to 10000 inhabitants living' at the elevations expressed in feet on the sides of the diagram.

The length of the *black horizontal lines* shows the *calculated* relative fatality of cholera in districts at relative elevations indicated by the height from the base of the diagram. The *dotted lines* indicate the mean mortality *observed* in the elevations given. Thus:—in districts at 90 feet above the Thames, the average mortality from cholera was 22 in 10000 inhabitants.

William S Farr's pyramid representing the cases of cholera by London suburb by the height of habitation during the 1849 cholera outbreak. Farr made the connection between mortality and lower elevation, but failed to connect lower elevation to poor drainage.

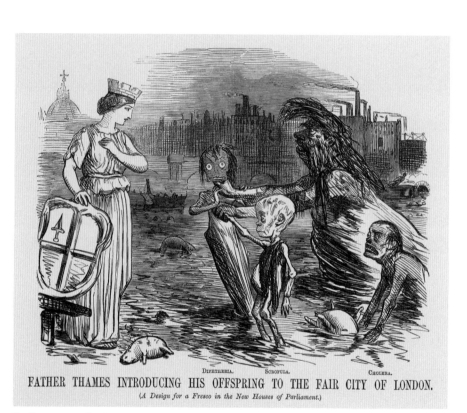

DIPHTHERIA.   SCROFULA.   CHOLERA.

FATHER THAMES INTRODUCING HIS OFFSPRING TO THE FAIR CITY OF LONDON.

(A Design for a Fresco in the New Houses of Parliament.)

By the summer of 1858 the 'Big Stink' had made it plain to many that the filthy river and the city's water supply were linked to cholera, scrofula and diptheria. *Punch*, July 3, 1858.

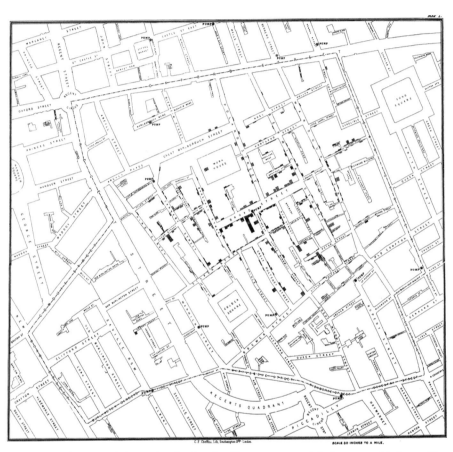

Snow's map of the 1854 cholera outbreak in London. The suspect pump is in the centre of the image. The workhouse is above it and the brewery to its right. With independent water supplies they did not use the pump and had no cases of cholera.

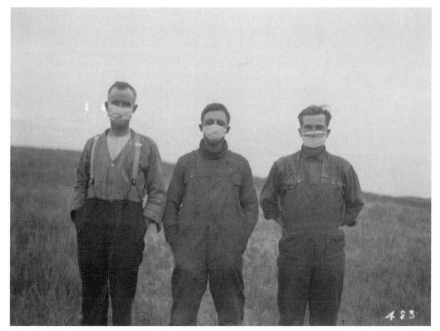

Three Canadian workers wearing masks during the 1918 influenza pandemic. It is an image that COVID-19 has made common in 2020.

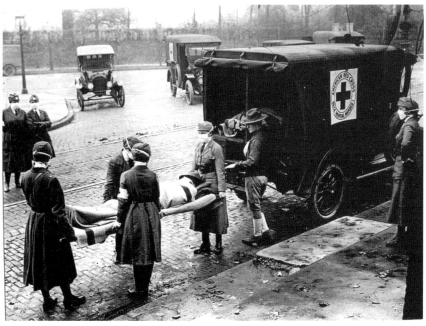

With masks over their faces, members of the American Red Cross remove a victim of the Spanish Flu from a house at Etzel and Page Avenues, St Louis, Missouri.

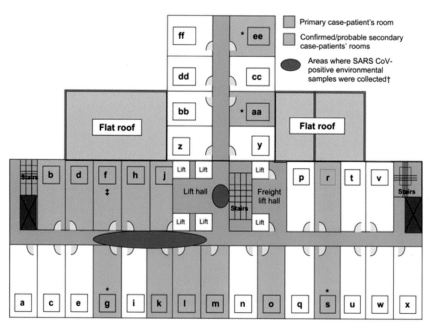

This diagram clearly shows how 'shared air' in the Metropole Hotel set the stage for a global pandemic. It travelled to Hong Kong from Guangdong and then on to Hong Kong, Toronto, Singapore and Vietnam.

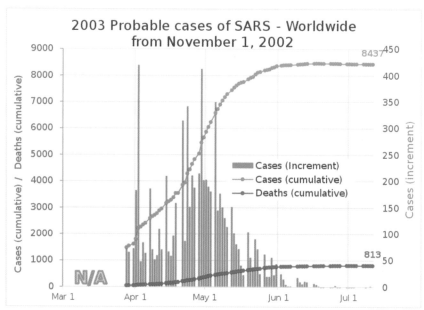

This graph displays the course of the 2003 SARS pandemic. It clearly demonstrates that mortality lags behind new infections and continues to rise even as new infections decline. Data source: Cumulative Number of Reported Probable Cases of Severe Acute Respiratory Syndrome (SARS).

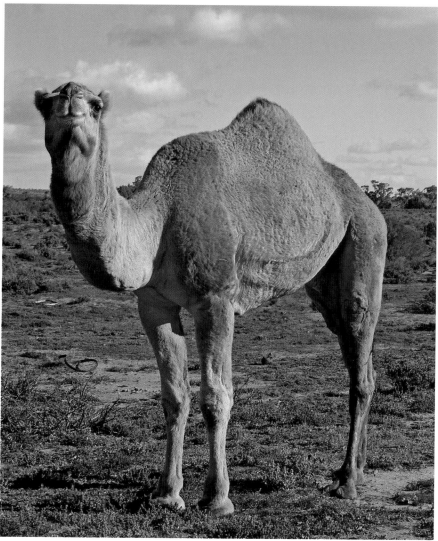

Dromedary camels are a major reservoir host for MERS-CoV and an animal source of MERS infection in humans. However, the exact role of dromedaries in transmission of the virus and the exact route(s) of transmission are unknown.

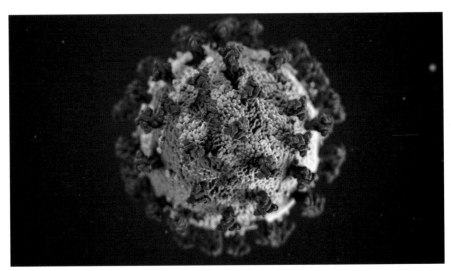

This illustration, created at the Centers for Disease Control and Prevention (CDC), reveals ultrastructural morphology exhibited by coronaviruses. Note the spikes that adorn the outer surface of the virus, which impart the look of a corona surrounding the virion, when viewed electron microscopically. A novel coronavirus, named Severe Acute Respiratory Syndrome coronavirus 2 (SARS-CoV-2), was identified as the cause of an outbreak of respiratory illness first detected in Wuhan, China in 2019. The illness caused by this virus has been named coronavirus disease 2019 (COVID-19).

4.

Cholera Pandemics

"A contagious disease we would define as one that is produced by a specific virus or morbid matter, that has either by contact or in the form of sweat – vapour from the breath – or some other excretion from the body, emanated from the sick of the disease, and which is capable of producing the same disease in another person. According to this definition, cholera is not contagious."

Dr Elam Stimson, *The Cholera Beacon*, 1835

SUGGESTIONS OF a cholera-like disease can be found in Sanskrit texts from the fifth century BCE and it has been endemic in the Indian subcontinent for centuries. Gaspar Correia, a Portuguese explorer, described in the *Lendas da India* (*Legends of India*) in 1543 an outbreak among army troops in Calicut and Goa to which 20,000 deaths were ascribed. He noted that the "disease (was characterised) by vomiting with drought of water accompanying it as if the stomach were parched up and cramps that force the sinews of the joints, disease sudden-like which struck with pain in the belly so that a man did not last out eight hours of time".

However, the first global pandemic did not erupt until 1817. It started in Jashore, in the Ganges delta, in August and then spread to Kolkata. It appeared in Cadiz in 1819 but did not gain a widespread foothold in Europe until 1830. It appeared in England, Scotland and Ireland the following year and crossed the Atlantic the next year. Subsequently, there were four more cholera pandemics throughout the 19th century and a sixth erupted in 1899.

Cholera is an acute secretory diarrhea caused by infection with the bacterium *Vibrio cholerae*. Ingested orally, the bacteria may be destroyed by gastric juices in the stomach. If the victim is malnourished or the intake of bacteria is excessive, some survives into the small intestine. There it attacks the mucous membrane lining the intestine. The small intestine is a semipermeable membrane. It allows nutrients to enter the body but does not transfer anything out of the body. Remarkably, the bacteria reverse this process: Nutrients stop passing into the body and blood plasma is drawn out of the victim, into the gastrointestinal system producing copious rice water diarrhea, toxic dehydration and, ultimately, death.

Eminent British physician Sir Thomas Watson told his students, "the malady was too striking to be overlooked, or ever forgotten, by one who had seen it." Unusually for a medical journal, *The Lancet* characterises it as "arresting": "Massive watery diarrhea, up to one litre per hour, can lead to hypotensive shock and death within hours of the first symptom (*cholera gravis*)... Although the stools of cholera patients may contain fecal matter or bile in the early phases, the characteristic 'rice water' stool of cholera develops with ongoing purging; this term refers to the similarity of the stool to water in which rice has been washed." The consequent severe dehydration had devastating effects. In 1893 cholera expert A. J. Wall wrote "In extreme cases, nearly the whole of the muscular system is affected – the calves, the thighs, the arms, the forearms, the muscles of the abdomen and back, the intercostal muscles, and those of the neck. The patient writhes in agony, and can scarcely be confined to his bed, his shrieks from this cause being very distressing to those around him." Voluminous, projectile diarrhea accompanied by vomiting, the first significant symptom of cholera, leads to rapid and fatal outcomes in the majority of cases if it is untreated.

Death can occur within hours of the onset of symptoms. A person could enjoy lunch with a friend and be dead by dinner. Passengers boarded trains healthy and died before arrival. People, literally, dropped dead in the streets. The case fatality rate approached 50%. And, in every case, the victims befouled themselves, their clothes, their caregivers' hands and their immediate environment with bacteria laden, rice water diarrhea.

Even the victim's corpse was horrifying, as well as infected. "A haunting feature of the disease is that it produces vigorous postmortem muscular contractions that cause limbs to shake and twitch for a prolonged period", Frank Snowden writes. "As a result, the death carts that collected the bodies of those who died of the disease seemed to be teeming with life, triggering fears of malevolent plots and of premature burial." The Victorian obsession with death is widely recognised; cholera's post-mortem animation of its victims mated with its rapid onset and high fatality rate marked it on the Victorian mind. According to Snowden, "it's not simply the body count that tells us how important a disease really is… Cholera, that had a limited body count, but a huge impact on civilisation." Yellow fever's 50,000 fatalities in Saint-Domingue, though small in the context of the tens of millions killed by the Black Death or Spanish flu, changed the history of a continent.

When *Vibrio cholerae* arrived in Europe and then North America in the early 19th century it encountered an ideal environment. It was in virgin soil for a new microbe, so resistance was nonexistent throughout the population. Further, increasing urbanisation and nascent industrialisation created a cluster of circumstances that together fostered cholera's spread. For the urban poor, housing was substandard and crowded, encouraging infection. An inadequate diet and endemic gastrointestinal infections meant malnutrition was widespread, impairing the immune system. Paramount was the simple fact that poor neighbourhoods in cities were disgusting, squalid, filthy messes. Most had nothing but a cesspit that human waste was dumped into. Sewers ran the gamut from primitive in big cities like London to nonexistent in colonial ports like Halifax, Nova Scotia. Potable water was not a municipal service and its availability was spotty and sketchy. In one famous instance, a community pump was located within three feet of a cesspit. In this situation it was inevitable that human waste tainted water supplies and infected the community.

Consequently, cholera epidemics followed a typical rhythm. Initially, it appeared in sporadic and isolated clusters focused on households, neighbourhoods and taverns or inns where food was served. These neighbourhoods generally shared two characteristics. First, they tended to be lower class. Second, they tended to be lower topographically, areas that liquid sewage would gravitate towards and accumulate in. It would often go unrecognised amid the gastrointestinal ailments then endemic – it was unlikely that its predominantly lower class victims would seek medical advice or be noticed by civic authorities. Inevitably infected human waste would eventually taint shallow wells and entered the water supply. Suddenly, an epidemic would erupt. With death often occurring in hours and a 50% fatality rate, mass casualties appeared almost instantaneously. Such was the predictable course of a cholera epidemic.

The disease moved from community to community aboard thoroughly modern conveniences according to the Constantinople International Sanitary Conference, 1866: "The Asiatic cholera, profiting, like man, from the modern discoveries, makes its incursions much easier than 50 years ago, and it spreads afar with all the rapidity of steamships and railway." Steamships provide the link to immigration. Immigrant ships were crowded and dirty. A single passenger boarding infected in Liverpool could lead to dozens of fatalities en route and a thoroughly infected ship arriving in New York or Halifax.

This first happened in British North America in 1832 and 1834. In the wake of these epidemics Elam Stimson published *The Cholera Beacon* in Dundas, Upper Canada (present day Ontario), in 1835. Dundas, nestled at the foot of the elbow of the Niagara Escarpment, was the westernmost point one could travel by water in British North America before the Welland Canal bypassed Niagara Falls. In the 1830s it was an important economic and transportation hub. As the site of the first paper mill in Upper Canada it was also home to G. H. Hackstaff, Publisher. A stopping off point for immigrants headed into western Upper Canada, it was hard hit in both the 1832 and 1834 epidemics. Today, it has been superceded by Hamilton Harbour and subsumed in the Regional Municipality of Hamilton-Wentworth. Surrounded by green space, development constrained by the escarpment, today it is an affluent, bucolic suburb.

The Cholera Beacon, "designed for popular instruction", offered a description of the "premonitory symptoms" and "directions for successful treatment" according to its monumental subtitle. Personally and professionally, Dr Stimson knew of which he wrote. Born in Connecticut, he studied medicine at Yale and then Dartmouth, graduating as class valedictorian in 1819. In 1823 he immigrated to St Catherines and then London, in Upper Canada. When cholera struck in 1832 he had a private practice in partnership with Dr James Corbin while serving as district coroner and physician to the town jail. Two years later he played a leading role in the London District when cholera struck again. He was a well-trained physician, by the standards of the era, who had practiced in Upper Canada for a dozen years, through two recent cholera epidemics. Professionally, he knew cholera as well as any physician in North America. He also knew the disease personally, having lost his wife and one of his children, a son, to it. For all of these reasons *The Cholera Beacon* provides an invaluable portrait of the medical understanding of the disease and its treatment in the 1830s.

Stimson was a firm believer in the miasma theory of cholera. Early on he declares that "surrounding the world, an impure state of the atmosphere exists, tending to produce cholera." Epidemics, 'local infections', usually erupt spontaneously "in the vicinity of great watercourses, and in low and marshy situations". In these locations epidemics are, "the product of heat and humidity, holding in solution a quantity of miasm, of exhalations of decaying animal or vegetable matter." In Upper Canada he referenced his home, London, at the forks of the Thames and the towns of Hamilton and Dundas, amid the marshlands at the 'Head of the Lake' – the western end of Lake Ontario. He made the topographical connection to 'low and marshy situations' but remained convinced it was airborne and naturally occurring, not water borne and reflective of poor sanitation and drainage.

He declares unequivocally and specifically that cholera is not infectious: "A contagious disease we would define as one that is produced by a specific virus or morbid matter, that has either by contact or in the form of sweat – vapour from the breath – or some other excretion from the body, emanated from the sick of the disease, and which is capable of producing the same disease in another person. According to this definition, Cholera is not contagious." He then goes on to elaborate on the miasma theory. Making the connection between infection and proximity to an infected person he states that the disease, particularly the malodorous diarrhea, "the filth incident to the

sick room", befouls the air, rendering "the epidemic influence more efficient."
It is for this reason also that he rejects traditional treatments for pandemics
such as burning fires juiced with pine tar and pitch, arguing that they impair
respiration and exacerbate the miasma's effects.

He states, without elaborating, that before a cholera outbreak, but with air
quality declining and the miasam growing stronger, "unusual morbid sensa-
tions are experienced by many persons, which have commonly been called
'premonitory symptoms'." While he hits the mark with "irregularity of the
bowels" the list is so long as to be meaningless, ranging from "fluttering of the
heart" to "frequent sighing". As the disease progresses he notes three types of
diarrhea that can occur before they converge into "a watery diarrhea... It is
now watery or very thin, and it passes from the body with little effort and a
sudden gush." He recalls patients saying, 'my insides were all in an uproar' and
'seems as if my bowels are all turning upside down'. Watery vomiting often
accompanies the diarrhea and signs of dehydration become evident including
a dry mouth and coated tongue, sunken eyes, thin cheeks and a raging thirst.
At this point, Stimson concedes the patient is beyond treatment and only a
handful who reach this stage will recover.

The Cholera Beacon then goes on to prescribe various treatments for cholera. Not surprisingly, bleeding, "three half pints or more" is recommended.
Doses of five grains each of calomel – a toxic solution of mercury chloride
– and capsicum alternating with peppermint, cloves or oregano oils in ginger
tea is also suggested. Clearly indicative of the paucity of medical interventions are the next set of recommendations, to be undertaken if the disease
worsens. They consist of nothing but more of the same, supplemented by
heat and massage. Particularly damaging would have been the bleeding: the
last thing a severely dehydrated patient needs is to have fluids removed, yet
Stimson advocates, "Draw blood – if it is thick and black and flows with
difficulty, only trickling slowly from the arm, the necessity of abstracting it is
great. Continue to draw blood (if you can) until it flows a full stream... If you
failed getting blood first, try again, and be sure to make a large opening in the
vein, even make an orifice in each arm." He, literally, tells practitioners to per-
severe because, "If you succeed in bleeding so as to cause it to flow freely and
become florid... a recovery may confidently be expected." The problem is that
a dehydrated cholera victim's blood will never 'flow freely and become florid.'

Beyond calomel and capsicum he also recommends a variety of potions standard in the Regency pharmacopeia such as Hiera Picra (aloe and canella, a cinnamon-like spice, tea), Huxham's Tincture and Elixir Proprietatus. The latter two consist of a variety of harmless, and equally ineffective, ingredients such as snakeroot, orange peel and Peruvian bark. These ingredients are dissolved in 60 ounces of whiskey and dispensed to the patient by the tablespoon multiple times daily. Throughout laudanum is recommended for pain when required. Unfortunately, this course of treatment, well intentioned and from a professional medical practitioner, based on the experience of two cholera epidemics, would have been ineffective.

Publishing a report from Liverpool, the Saint John's *Morning News* announced an 'infallible' remedy so accessible and simple as to "relieve all apprehensions of fatal results", certainly a backhanded guarantee. The elixir consisted of nothing more than a tablespoon of common salt and one of red pepper taken in hot water. The *Morning News* assured readers, "*The New York Times* has heard innumerable instances of its use, and not one of its failure." All of these futile rostrums, potions and practices were misdirected and reflected the glacial pace of change in medical science. Hippocrates, Galen and humoural medicine insisted with absolute certainty that cholera, like all pandemics, was miasmatic.

The contagious alternative was ridiculed by the New York *Constellation*'s reference to, "little, infernal, greedy, choleric *critters*." A handful of observers clung to astrological events disturbing the atmosphere, most commonly comets although one attributed cholera to a "moving non-electric meteor." Future Upper Canadian rebel leader, WIlliam Lyon Mackenzie was a miasmatist. In *Sketches of Canada and the United States* (1833) he reports that during the 1832 cholera epidemic in Montreal an experiment was undertaken that proved the miasmatic theory: a piece of "fresh wholesome beef was placed on the top of one of the Catholic new cathedral church spires, and taken down after an hour and 20 minutes, in a tainted and corrupt state." Ergo, the atmosphere itself was capable of causing degeneration and disease. Another miasma theory devotee, landscape architect Frederick Law Olmsted, advocated for the healing powers of parks, which he believed could act like urban lungs as "outlets for foul air and inlets for pure air."

American physician William Beaumont attributed mortality not to cholera, but rather, fear of cholera. "The greater proportional number of deaths in the cholera epidemics are, in my opinion, caused more by fright and presentiment of death than from the fatal tendency of the disease." This parallels Defoe's remark that some were frighted to death. In 1838 Sylvester Graham even explained how and why fear of cholera was fatal, "it spasmodically contracts the mouths of thousands of our perspiring or exhaling vessels, flings the acrid perspirable matter upon the insides of our digestive organs, which it stimulates, and causes by abstracting much of the watery part of our blood, a looseness and congestion in our bowels, the very proximate cause of the epidemic cholera." Elaborate though it is, it is wildly inaccurate. When cholera first appeared, medical science was at a loss.

In the face of medical failure, appeals to the Almighty endured. In his famous memoir, Frederick Douglass wrote, concerning 1832, "The cholera was on its way, and the thought was present, that God was angry with the white people because of their slaveholding wickedness, and, therefore, his judgments were abroad in the land. It was impossible for me not to hope much from the abolition movement, when I saw it supported by the Almighty, and armed with DEATH!" Scapegoating 'white people' certainly turns the tables on the traditional images of post-plague patsies.

And so too in 1834 in Halifax, "The Lieutenant Governor taking into consideration the danger with which the province is threatened by the progress of a grievous disease, have resolved, and do, by and with the advice of His Majesty's Council, hereby command a public day for fasting and humiliation be observed on Wednesday the 17th day of the present month of September." The order explicitly blamed the plague on divine displeasure with human behaviour: "that we may all humble ourselves before Almighty God, in order to obtain pardon for our sins and in the most devout and solemn manner send up our prayers and supplications to the Divine Majesty for averting those heavy judgments which our manifold provocations have most justly deserved, and particularly beseeching God to remove from us that grievous disease." In the 1830s miasma caused cholera and an appeal to the divine was entirely reasonable with medical science straitjacketed by humouralism.

By 1832 Halifax had been dealing with immigrant ships, occasionally bearing disease-ridden human cargo since its inception. In recent years typhus and yellow fever led the list. In September 1827, the immigrant brig *James* entered Halifax harbour from Saint John's. Leaving Dublin, its destination was Quebec City. It had been forced to stop in St John's; 35 passengers were too ill to continue and five had been buried at sea en route. Leaving Newfoundland for Quebec City it made for Halifax when typhus broke out again. Upon its arrival on September 7, flying the yellow jack, indicating epidemic disease aboard, Nova Scotia's Lieutenant-Governor James Kempt was furious. He wrote to the Prime Minister, Viscount Goderich, "There arrived this day in the brig James from Waterford 120 passengers of the most wretched description, all of whom, as well as the whole crew... are labouring under typhus fever." He blamed "scanty nourishment during the voyage... the crowded and filthy state of the ship and... a want of medical assistance." He added, "I wish that this were the only case of a like nature that I could adduce," but that five other infected arrivals had preceded it that summer.

Typhus ultimately claimed 800 of 12,000 Haligonians (7%) that year. Kempt argued that the young colony could not afford the burden and strongly hinted that the British had an obligation to ensure that infected vessels and immigrants were not allowed to depart British ports. This was reinforced by a report in November from the council predicting a catastrophe and demanding legislative intervention, "Under these circumstances disease is inevitable... The law which restrained these evils is no longer in force in Great Britain, and we have no legislative enactment there to prevent the recurrence of the calamity which we have endured this year, or to punish the authors of it." Nova Scotia's interests were overridden by Imperial demands. In the wake of the Napoleonic Wars, Britain underwent severe long term under employment and emigration became an inexpensive and effective way to shovel out the poor.

In 1832, when cholera arrived in British North America, Quebec City lost 10% of its population and Montréal 15%. From there it spread west into Upper Canada, notably its largest city, York (Toronto). From Upper Canada it spread back east through the United States along the Erie Canal and from Lower Canada south through Lake Champlain to New York City.

Halifax undertook extensive, and expensive, preparations for epidemic diseases. In 1827 an emigrant hospital had been built, and in 1831 a smallpox hospital was constructed on Melville Island to isolate infected emigrants.

In 1832, three additional hospitals staffed by two doctors and a physician's assistant were also prepared. Then the city was spared, despite a regular flow of immigrants not a single case was reported. It was held up as an example of a city that 'warded off' cholera. The attribution of agency was unjustified; the port simply avoided cholera rather than warding it off. It was good luck rather than good management that spared Halifax.

In 1834 cholera ravaged the city, killing 400. A parsimonious (and self-satisfied) government prevaricated and scrimped on preparations. In the first week of August both the *Acadian Recorder* and the *Novascotian* reported deaths from cholera in Lower Canada. The latter noted, "Canadian papers do not say more about it than they can help." On August 13 the *Novascotian* noted rumours of cholera deaths in the Halifax poorhouse, and a categorical denial from the Board of Health. On the 23rd, official denials were abrogated by the *Recorder* reporting cholera in the poorhouse, among the garrison, and throughout the city. By the 30th, 35 members of the garrison had died and the *Recorder* was asking why, "The military are supposed to be kept clean, well clothed, and regularly fed. These particulars are acknowledged preventatives of cholera, why then, according to the nature of things, should those enjoying them be selected as victims?"

The *Novascotian* argued that not enough had been spent on preparations because too much had been wasted two years earlier: "Two years ago the most ample preparation was made and very heavy expenses incurred, for the reception of cholera, but the cholera did not come... It is probable enough that the whole thing might have been managed with more economy; and if anybody could have foreseen that the disease would have been two years travelling from Canada here, several thousands might have been saved." This is a straw man argument. Nobody 'could have foreseen that the disease would have been two years travelling from Canada'. Ample preparations for the 1832 epidemic were no prophylactic two years later. This balancing act between the cost of preparing for a pandemic and the likelihood of one occurring is a timeless problem for bureaucrats and politicians. It was summed up by George W. Bush's secretary of Health and Human Services, Michael Leavitt: "In advance of a pandemic, anything you say sounds alarmist, after a pandemic starts, everything you've done is inadequate."

Later in 1834 the Colonial Office granted Lieutenant-Governor Campbell £500 for extraordinary immigrant related epidemic expenses. The lieutenant-governor estimated that to be only one-third of the costs of the epidemic and responded by sending more than 75 impoverished English back, evoking fury in the Colonial Office.

Three decades later, while the British North American colonies debated Confederation, cholera struck Halifax again. At 4898 tons, SS *England*, a 420hp, steamship built in 1865, was owned by the National Line, a Liverpool based consortium. On her maiden voyage she left Liverpool on Wednesday, March 28, 1866, stopping at Queenstown (in County Cork, southern Ireland, known as the 'Cove of Cork' before 1849 and since 1922 as Cobh) to pick up passengers before heading on to New York. The 1200 in steerage were German immigrants who boarded in Liverpool and Irish immigrants who boarded in Queenstown. There were two dozen saloon passengers. The *England* arrived in Queenstown a day later, and after boarding all the new passengers, she sailed later that night.

Cholera broke out after a three-day gale that caused the steerage passengers to be battened down below decks. Needless to add, with fecal-oral transmission, this would have been a bonanza for *Vibrio cholerae*. Family oral histories recall the mortality rate skyrocketing. "Four days later, an eight-year-old German boy was found dead in his bed from cholera. The next morning, another passenger, Thomas Walsh, aged 35, died… The next day ten died; the following day 50 died, and so on." The ship headed for Halifax where it dropped anchor in the bay and raised the yellow jack on April 9.

That evening Mayor Mathew Henry Richey gaveled the regular Halifax City Council meeting to order. The Sanitary Committee reported on its inspection of slaughterhouses. They produced a list of abattoirs that should be licensed and recommended that all future slaughterhouses require approval by the committee. Again, the concern was the malodorous effluvia not the water supply. The city clerk was directed to summon the proprietor of the Horse Railway to appear before council, "for placing a nuisance in Upper Water Street and other streets and not removing the same within the time allowed by law." Finally, it was decided to advertise for the position of Clerk of Streets until the 20th day of April. By then these workaday concerns would be long forgotten. The *England* had been directed to the quarantine station on McNabb's Island. King Cholera had come to visit Halifax again.

By the time the city council next met on Monday, April 21, the first order of business would be a letter of condolences to a widow. This was the widow of Dr John Slayter, Halifax Officer of Health, who was already dead of the cholera he contracted from patients he was tending at the quarantine station. The quarantined were housed in tents; their belongings were burned and, although they were given new clothing, blankets and provisions, violence broke out and both police and troops had to be ordered to the island to maintain order. Labourers had to be dispatched to bury the dead in the cemetery at the south end of the island. The *England* was cleaned and fumigated. On April 18, she left Halifax for New York (carrying cholera aboard still). Some of the passengers were left behind on McNab's Island. They departed Halifax on May 17 and arrived in New York on May 24, 1866.

Again, quarantine was well intentioned but ineffective. It was misdirected because it was designed to quarantine the miasmatic effusions of the infected. In fact, there were various routes by which the disease could travel from the quarantine station to the city. Residents passing back and forth – from gravediggers and policemen to doctors – posed the most obvious threat. Laundresses washing the clothes and bedding of infected ship's crews and passengers were at risk. So were scavengers who collected bedding discarded from infected ships. Harbourfront inns and taverns that served food were problematic. Finally, and unusually, seafood itself was a vector. Benthic crustaceans such as crabs and lobsters, and bivalves including clams and scallops, are bottom feeders. Human fecal material from infected ships in the harbour settled on the seafloor, was consumed by the local wildlife and infected it. Anyone eating these creatures, unless they were thoroughly cooked, would become infected.

With all these avenues of infection and the misdirected emphasis on miasma, Haligonians' practical efforts to deal with cholera were largely ineffective. The same can be said of other cities. Even the most rigorous sanitation programmes were directed at reducing odours rather than preventing the contamination of drinking water.

Beneath the surface, a tectonic shift was taking place. The behemoth of humouralism was under assault, but it would not go easily despite the mounting evidence that it was dead wrong. Historian of science Thomas Kuhn coined the term paradigm shift over 50 years ago, referencing the Copernican Revolution. Once upon a time, the sun revolved around the earth, yet after Copernicus the earth revolved around the sun in the company of other planets. At a stroke, everything was turned upside down. One fundamental revelation and the entire universe was changed. A paradigm shift is considerably more than a change of method or mood; everything changes. After two millennia, humouralism was about to be cast aside in what amounted to the blink of an eye in historical terms, a mere half century.

Between 1849 and 1854, London physician John Snow proposed that cholera was a communicable disease and that stool contained infectious material. He suggested that this infectious material could contaminate drinking water supplies, resulting in transmission of cholera. A leading anesthesiologist of his era, his practice included administering chloroform to Queen Victoria during the birth of her last two children. In 1849, during a cholera epidemic, he published *On the Mode of Communication of Cholera*. More than a decade before the germ theory was developed by Louis Pasteur, Snow proposed that cholera was centered in the gastro-intestinal system and its "ejections and dejections" contaminated the infected and their bedding, the hands of their caregivers and, ultimately, neighbouring wells and water supplies. This assertion directly contradicted the miasma theory of disease by dismissing infected air and identifying a vector for community spread. Snow correctly pointed out that a caregiver with dirty hands, most frequently female, might then prepare a meal and spread the infection throughout the family. His reputation gave weight to his revolutionary proposals and in the following year he was admitted to the Royal College of Physicians and a founding member of the Epidemiological Society of London.

At the time, water was not a public service and was provided by private companies with parallel supply networks and separate sources. Many residents and businesses still relied on private wells. In 1854, the Lambeth Waterworks Company had just moved its source 22 miles upstream of London, preempting London's effluvia, while the Southwark and Vauxhall Water Company continued to draw its supply from the Thames in the heart of the city. It was an experiment waiting to happen and Snow made it so. He drew out statistical evidence of his theory, again, before germ theory was circulating.

In a pioneering work of medical mapping, he linked a particularly virulent outbreak in Soho to a specific community water pump on Broad Street. An adjacent workhouse with 500 inmates had only five cases and a neighbouring brewery seemed immune. Not coincidentally, each had its own well and did not draw water from the community pump. Moreover, when Snow had the pump handle removed, decommissioning it, infections evaporated. Not surprisingly, the Broad Street pump was supplied by the Southwark and Vauxhall Water Company.

Simultaneously, Tuscan doctor Filippo Pacini, an early microscopist and professor of medicine at the University of Florence, working independently in Italy in 1854, first observed comma-shaped forms under a microscope in cholera stools. He labelled them *Vibrio* and his work was promptly forgotten. Thirty years later, German Robert Koch first isolated *V. cholerae* in pure culture in work that began in Egypt and continued in Calcutta (Kolkata), India. However, this is not to suggest that the miasma theory was suddenly eliminated. It persisted throughout the century. As late as 1874, at the International Sanitary Conference convened in Vienna, representatives of 21 governments voted unanimously that "ambient air is the principal vehicle of the generative agent of cholera." A year later, in Brussels the Conference conceded that air *and* water could transmit cholera. This resistance to mounting evidence that contradicts the established paradigm is known as the Semmelweiss reflex. In 1847, Hungarian physician Ignaz Semmelweiss realised that puerperal fever could be reduced by hand washing between patients, and particularly between autopsy cadavers and patients, to prevent transmission of "cadaverous particles." Despite the plain evidence, hand hygiene was dismissed as irrelevant or unnecessary. Early suggestions that cholera was waterborne not miasmatic met with the same knee jerk dismissal.

Tragically, early experiments with the only method available at the time that might have helped cholera victims, intravenous rehydration, was similarly laughed out of the academy. Humouralism held that the physician should facilitate the body's natural impulses and bleed and administer emetics to further evacuations and encourage the cholera patient's attempts to expel fluids. Directly contrary to prevailing medical theory and practice, building on the work of doctors William O'Shaughnessy and William Stevens, Dr Thomas Aitchison Latta (c. 1796-1833) experimented with intravenous saline rehydration during the first cholera pandemic in 1832, when rehydration rectally failed, "Having inserted a tube into the basilic vein, cautiously – anxiously, I watched the effects; ounce after ounce was injected, but no visible change was produced. Still persevering, I thought she began to breathe less laboriously, soon the sharpened features, and sunken eye, and fallen jaw, pale and cold, bearing the manifest impress of death's signet, began to glow with returning animation; the pulse, which had long ceased, returned to the wrist; at first small and quick, by degrees it became more and more distinct." Despite clinical success, *The Lancet*, firmly humouralist, ridiculed the method – "the most trumpery book for its size that it has fallen our lot to review" – and it was 70 years before the practice was revived. Today, it is the first priority for physicians treating cholera.

Despite resistance to the idea that cholera was waterborne, miasmatists believed that cesspits, abattoirs and dirty, standing water were linked to cholera as sources of miasma. Throughout the 19th century, reactions to pandemics focused on the right issue – sanitation – for the wrong reasons, reducing sources of miasma. In 1858, a drought caused a precipitous drop in the level of the Thames in London, exposing the riverbed along the banks. It caused the 'Great Stink', an odour so repugnant it forced the closure of the Houses of Parliament and the construction of a modern sewer system that transported the city's waste far enough away from London that the river's tides did not wash it back upstream into the city water supply. In addition, the muddy shorelines of the Thames were narrowed and replaced with the famous Embankment with riverside roads and gardens.

Across the English Channel, Emperor Napoleon III came to power in France in 1848 amid a cholera outbreak that took the lives of approximately 19,000 Parisians. This left him determined to redesign Paris salubriously, "Let us open new streets, make the working class quarters, which lack air and light, more healthy, and let the beneficial sunlight reach everywhere within our walls," he declared. To this end, Baron Georges-Eugène Haussmann demolished 12,000 buildings and replaced them with tree-lined boulevards, fountains, parks and, most importantly, an elaborate sewage system that transformed Paris. Planning for Frederick Law Olmsted's Central Park began in the immediate aftermath of New York's second cholera outbreak.

Thanks to the success of that project, Olmsted, whose first child had died of cholera, went on to design more than 100 public parks and recreation grounds including those in Boston, Buffalo, Chicago and Detroit. These changes culminated in the 'City Beautiful' movement at the end of the century, with its emphasis on greenery, natural spaces, sunlight and fresh air. Coupled with municipal water treatment and improved sanitation the dual scourges of dysentery and cholera were largely eliminated from North America and Europe by the end of the 19th century.

Repeated cholera outbreaks throughout the 19th century had few significant economic, political or diplomatic consequences. However, they had earth-shaking medical and public health consequences. Paramount was the death of miasmatism and acceptance that cholera involved oral-fecal transmission: a paradigm shift in medical thought. In terms of practical public health, cholera inspired an interest in civic works to improve sewage and drainage. Even miasmatists supported this as they believed the odours from human waste and polluted water tainted the air and were infectious. Ironically, the first pandemic of the 20th century would turn out to be influenza, a virus that is transmitted through the air.

5.

Influenza: The First Modern Epidemic

"If the epidemic continues its mathematical rate of acceleration, civilisation could easily disappear from the face of the earth within a few weeks."

Col. Victor C. Vaughan, Director, Communicable
Diseases Division, US Army (1918-1919);
Dean, U of Michigan Medical School (1891-1921);
President, AMA (1914-1915)

IN THE summer of 1914 the European powers, ensnared in their own web of alliances, stumbled into the world's first modern, global war. A Bosnian terrorist murdered the heir to the Austro-Hungarian Empire; Serbia was blamed and threatened by Austria-Hungary; Russia mobilised to defend Serbia, its Slav ally. This obliged Germany to mobilise to defend its Austro-Hungarian partner, triggering French mobilisation and drawing England into the war too. It was the world's first industrial, mass production war.

Machine guns and artillery displaced sabres and steeds. Aircraft, poison gas and submarines were added to the witches' brew. For the next four years the fire burned and the cauldron bubbled but the trench lines in western Europe remained stubbornly fixed. In the spring of 1918 Germany launched a massive offensive hoping to decide the struggle before American troops began flooding into France. It failed, and an Allied counteroffensive in August initiated the 'Hundred Days' victory campaign that culminated in the Armistice on November 11. Coincident to the conclusion of this first modern war the world was enduring its first modern pandemic.

The scope of the 1918-1919 influenza pandemic (subtype H1N1) boggles the imagination. It was, and remains, the deadliest disease outbreak in human history. Almost one-third of the globe's population was infected and probably close to 100 million died over three years, most between September 1918 and March 1919. In the developed world, the overall mortality was about 2%: A quarter of a million in the UK, 675,000 in the USA and 55,000 in Canada died. The vast majority of infections and deaths, and the lion's share of the suffering, occurred outside North America and Europe.

India and China are both thought to have suffered around 20 million deaths. By way of comparison, in 2019 it is estimated that 400,000 people died of influenza globally, roughly one flu death per 20,000. During the flu pandemic the rate was one flu death per 100 persons in the world, roughly 200 times higher. Unusually, half of those infected were healthy young men and women under 40. Even famous German soldier Ernst Jünger took note of this phenomenon, "Young men in particular sometimes died overnight." This overall data neglects regional variations and the course of the pandemic over time, but these gross numbers are, literally, gross. In total, fatalities from the influenza pandemic exceeded the Black Death.

The influenza epidemic swept over the globe in three successive waves. The first, erupting in Kansas in the spring of 1918, was relatively mild and mistaken by many for a bad, but not atypical, seasonal flu. In August it became noticeable in western Europe and the Eastern Seaboard of the United States. The second and deadliest wave swept across the United States from east to west in the final three months of 1918. In Philadelphia and Boston it leapt from military personnel to civilians. Troop movements and civilians using roads and rail carried the virus westward. In October 1918, 195,000 American deaths were attributable to the flu pandemic. The most virulent wave of the virus was peaking as the United States held mid-term elections on Tuesday, November 5, and 'the War to End All Wars' ended on

Monday, November 11, 1918. At the same time the pandemic spread globally, emerging in Brazil, South Africa, India and China. Australia (but not New Zealand) and American Samoa (but not Western Samoa) were two of the few places to escape the virus. A light third wave, some regard it as an 'echo' of the second wave, occurred in the first months of 1919.

The flu pandemic can, literally and legitimately, lay claim to the title of 'mother' of all flu pandemics. As American microbiologists Jeffery K. Taubenberger and David M. Morens explain, "Almost all cases of influenza A worldwide (excepting human infections from avian viruses such as H5N1 and H7N7), have been caused by descendants of the 1918 virus, including 'drifted' H1N1 viruses and re-assorted H2N2 and H3N2 viruses … composed of key genes from the 1918 virus, updated by subsequently incorporated avian influenza genes that code for novel surface proteins, making the 1918 virus indeed the 'mother' of all pandemics."

The H in a flu designation refers to the antigen Haemagglutinin, the spike on a virus that penetrates the human cell allowing the virus to insert its RNA. In flu nomenclature N refers to Neuraminidase, the antigen that allows the multiplying viruses to break out of the host cell. Viruses, containing only RNA, are notoriously labile. Minor changes known as drift occur frequently and explain the need for an updated flu vaccine annually. Periodically new A strains of flu emerge and cause pandemics, H2 in 1957 and H3 in 1968. Finally, if a host is infected by multiple viruses their reproduction can become mixed, leading to 'shift' or re-assortment to a novel H-N combination.

The 1918-19 influenza pandemic is the first documented H1 pandemic, the entire globe was virgin soil for this mother of influenza pandemics. However, all of this information has only emerged in this century. Viruses were suspected in 1918 but unknown; they were too small to be seen until the electron microscope was invented in the 1930s. In 1918 doctors believed that influenza was bacterial not viral, a fundamental error that undermined efforts to treat the disease.

This pandemic has deliberately not been referred to by its common label, the 'Spanish Flu. The Spanish flu had nothing to do with Spain. It did not originate in Spain and Spain was not particularly severely affected. The Spanish have suffered eponymously for their honesty and diplomacy.

Diplomatically, Spain dodged a bullet by staying neutral during the First World War (a balancing act it was able to repeat during the second).

The combatants regarded information about the pandemic as a potential threat to their war fighting ability and a national security issue. On both sides of the trenches, they worried that news of the pandemic would give succour to the enemy. Consequently, during the early stages of the outbreak reporting on the pandemic was suppressed and censored in the warring nations. The Spanish press faced no such restrictions and freely reported on the alarming spread of deadly influenza. Nothing less than the accuracy of Spanish journalists and the transparency of their government has hung the handle Spanish flu on the nation.

As a warning to the wise, the Spanish flu probably made its zoonotic leap from swine to human in the heart of the United States; consequently, if it deserves a geographic label, it is the 'Kansas Flu', the 'Sunflower State Flu' or the 'American Flu'. Regardless, throughout it will be referred to as simply the influenza pandemic. That said there are two competing theories as to its origins that also merit mention. Canadian military historian Mark Humphries traces the first outbreak to the Chinese Labour Corps (CLC) – arguing that they brought it to the Western Front from Shansi province, where a late fall 1917 epidemic killed 16,000. The problem with this theory is that there is no evidence as to precisely what the epidemic in Shansi was nor how it made it to Kansas so quickly.

Another theory ties it to a flu outbreak in December 1916 at the massive British base at Étaples, south of Boulogne-sur-Mer. *The Lancet* labelled it "purulent [discharging pus] bronchitis", noted the victims' lungs were severely congested and inflamed, that oxygen deprivation gave a blueish tint to the skin (symptoms of the subsequent pandemic) and linked it to patients whose lungs had been previously weakened by poison gas. Similar outbreaks occurred in the British military hospital at Rouen and Aldershot Barracks in Hampshire. According to this theory the virus made the leap to humans from waterfowl, primarily ducks. The Somme estuary is only 30 miles north of Étaples and a major stopover for migrating waterfowl. Recent research has identified hundreds of flu viruses in the duck population that pass by. However, if this was a precursor of the flu pandemic one has to wonder where and why it disappeared for 16 months until the spring of 1918.

The theory that dominates the field traces the outbreak to Haskell County, Kansas. American historian John M. Barry writes simply, "If the virus did not originate in Haskell, there is no good explanation for how it arrived there. There were no other known outbreaks anywhere in the United States from which someone could have carried the disease to Haskell and no suggestions of influenza outbreaks in either newspapers or reflected in vital statistics anywhere else in the region". In the words of Sherlock Holmes, "when you have eliminated the impossible, whatever remains, however improbable, must be the truth". Haskell County was rural and poor; sod houses and living with the livestock poor. A flu so severe that a Haskell County doctor, Loring Miner, reported it to the US Public Health Service broke out in January 1918. Weeks later draftees from Haskell County arrived at Camp Funston, part of 100,000 acre Fort Riley, 100 miles west of Kansas City.

There on the morning of Tuesday, March 4, Private Albert Gitchell reported at sick call, complaining of sore throat, fever and headache. By noon, 107 of his comrades were complaining of similar symptoms. An influenza outbreak was under way. Outbreaks followed throughout the military, in prisons and across the country. Five weeks later, more than 1000 soldiers had been infected and 47 were dead. It had become an influenza pandemic. America had entered the war one year earlier and the pandemic's arrival coincided with a massive movement of American soldiers to France. Between this first case and the end of April more than 200,000 American soldiers were shipped to Europe, carrying the influenza virus with them. A year later, the retrograde movement, the demobilisation of soldiers and their return home, would again carry the virus far and wide to even the most remote corners of the combatants' homelands.

Writing at the time Dr David J. Payne, believed this new influenza was distinctive. Uniquely, "it produced a deep cyanosis (blue skin) and a bluish froth around the nose and the mouth – the so-called heliotrope cyanosis – culminating with the horrific drowning of the victim in his (her) own body fluids. There was also an extraordinarily high mortality rate of 20 times the norm for influenza. Death often occurred within a few hours. In many of the cases that did survive the critical first few days of the influenza attack, death was precipitated by a rampant secondary infection by pneumonia bacteria." Weakened by influenza, immediate cause of death was often pneumonia. The

Spanish flu hit the world in the days before antibiotics were invented; and many deaths, perhaps most, were not caused by the influenza virus itself, but resulted directly from secondary bacterial pneumonia caused by common upper respiratory tract bacteria. This was rare for seasonal influenza, and complicates statistical accounting: did a fatality die of pneumonia as the direct cause of death or did they die of influenza because it rendered them unable to resist pneumonia?

Working in the base hospital at Camp Devens, near Boston, during the vicious second wave of the flu, physician Roy Grist wrote, "These men start with what appears to be an ordinary attack of LaGrippe or influenza, and when brought to the hosp. they very rapidly develop the most vicious type of pneumonia that has ever been seen. Two hours after admission they have the mahogany spots over the cheek bones, and a few hours later you can begin to see the cyanosis extending from their ears and spreading all over the face... It is only a matter of a few hours then until death comes."

The symptoms he describes are now known as a cytokine storm. In the face of influenza, possibly complicated by pneumonia, sensing it is being overwhelmed, the body's immune system launches an all out response so extreme it attacks everything, viral or not, and literally destroys the lungs. The destruction, according to the noted influenza expert Edwin Kilbourne, resembled nothing so much as the lesions from "the inhalation of poison gas". A similar response has been seen among some COVID-19 patients. These cytokine storms may explain the unusual mortality profile of the 1918-19 pandemic. Young people, with stronger immune systems, may have been more likely to deploy cytokine storms in response to influenza, and fallen victim to their very immune systems. Another explanation may also be a factor. If the 1889-92 flu pandemic was an ancestor of the 1918-19 pandemic, older people alive during the earlier pandemic may have had some resistance or immunity that younger people did not.

On the other hand, the earlier flu pandemic wrong footed medical science in a particularly damaging way. During the 1889-1892 pandemic German physician Richard Pfeiffer had isolated bacteria from influenza patients and wrongly believed that these bacteria were the cause of influenza; the bacteria had come to be known as *Pfeiffer's bacillus* or *Bacillus influenzae* and a vaccine was developed. In the 19th century diphtheria, typhus and cholera were all bacterial infections. It made sense to assume influenza was bacterial, particularly with viruses as yet unseen and undiscovered. However, influenza is a respiratory virus, it is not a bacteria. Doctors at the time did not know what they were dealing with. It was a case of mistaken identity.

The *Journal of the American Medical Association* editorialised, "There is, therefore, no basis on which promise of protection from vaccines may be made. They may be harmless, and they may or may not be of preventive value." In Canada, Director-General of Public Health, Dr P. Montizambert opined that even an ineffective vaccine would have positive mental effects, "There is of course a further psychological value, either greater or smaller, in the effect of a harmless vaccine, in giving confidence to those who have to be exposed to infection and preventing panic on the part of others, just as the lump of camphor worn round the neck or potato carried in the pocket for rheumatism, the mind acting on the body and enhancing its powers of resistance."

This groping in the dark led to the bizarre saga that is Aspirin's link to the influenza pandemic. In 1900 the German firm Bayer received a patent for Acetyl Salicylic Acid 2 and marketed it under the brand name Aspirin. In 1917, Bayer, now an enemy firm, lost its proprietary rights and Aspirin went generic. It was inexpensive and widely available. In 1918, the US Surgeon General, the US Navy and the *Journal of the American Medical Association* all advocated mega-doses of Aspirin for patients. One memoir recalls Aspirin being given "by the half-handful over and over". More precisely, recommended dosages ranged from 8g to 31.2g per day. Today these are recognised as toxic, even fatal doses. According to Dr Karen Starko, these dosages "produce levels associated with hyperventilation and pulmonary edema in 33% and 3% of recipients, respectively. Recently, pulmonary edema was found at autopsy in 46% of 26 salicylate-intoxicated adults." When not fatal they magnify influenza's symptoms because they "increase lung fluid and protein levels and impair mucociliary clearance." The treatment was killing patients. Starko concludes, "In summary, just before the 1918 death spike, aspirin was recommended in regimens now known to be potentially toxic and to cause pulmonary edema and may therefore have contributed to overall pandemic mortality and several of its mysteries. Young adult mortality may be explained by willingness to use the new, recommended therapy and the presence of youth in regimented treatment settings (military)." The Aspirin regimen was contributing to the death toll in the United States, particularly among the young.

At the same time as the government was recommending Aspirin, rumours were circulating on the Eastern seaboard that Bayer was tainting Aspirin with influenza bacteria and the entire pandemic was a German biological attack. In a classic case of pandemic behaviour the rumour that Aspirin was responsible for influenza deaths was a typical case of scapegoating. Ironically, it was right for all the wrong reasons. The medication was not tainted yet it was responsible for killing influenza patients, albeit thanks to America's own physicians.

Experiments were also made with transfusions of blood serum from convalescent patients for the first time. It met with notable success and the Surgeon General of the US Navy reported, "The cases treated with serum showed striking and immediate improvement clinically in most instances" and the CFR declined from approximately 25% to 6%. Although the pandemic ended before this treatment was widespread, it has been one of many methods investigated for the treatment of COVID-19.

There is also a certain medical irony to the situation. For millennia the humoural school attributed pandemics to infected air. Over the course of the 19th century the discovery that cholera was waterborne and Walter Reed's demonstration that mosquitoes carried yellow fever debunked the theory of miasma. Yet, as history would have it the first pandemic of the 20th century was, in fact, airborne.

At the height of the influenza pandemic the American Public Health Association admitted, "in the face of the greatest pestilence that ever struck this country we are just as ignorant as the Florentine were with the plague described in history." With medical science stymied shysters, hucksters and shills were ever ready to offer cures and profit from the fear of infection. Dr Franklin Duane gave interviews and ran advertisements attesting to the prophylactic value of "Dr Pierce's Pleasant Pellets". Dr Bell's Pine Tar Honey, Schenck's Mandrake Pills, Beecham's Pills and Miller's Antiseptic Snake Oil also promised protection or relief from the flu. Users were assured that, "When [Vick's] VapoRub is applied over the throat and chest, the medicated vapors loosen the phlegm, open the air passages and stimulate the mucus membrane to throw off the germs." In an age of patent medicines a pandemic was a marketers' dream come true.

Folk treatments popped up as people were desperate for protection. One was wearing camphor balls in a sack around the neck. It was believed the pungent odour would purify the air around the wearer; an approach that echoes 'a pocketful of posies' and the plague doctor's beak filled with aromatics. *The News of the World* offered a variety of measures readers should take: "Wash inside nose with soap and water each night and morning; force yourself to sneeze night and morning, then breathe deeply; do not wear a muffler; take sharp walks regularly and walk home from work; eat plenty of porridge." These nostrums were, at least harmless, and walking home from work, implying avoiding public transit, was sound advice.

Certain groups demonstrated elevated mortality. For instance, a Metropolitan Life Insurance Company study of people aged 25 to 45 found that 3.26% of all industrial workers and 6% of all coal miners died. Elevated levels for the latter group was probably linked to their coal dust laden and close quarter working environment with extremely poor ventilation. In a similar manner, researchers have linked elevated COVID-19 deaths to locales with high levels of air pollution. Other studies found that for pregnant women, fatality rates ranged from 23% to 71% which is astonishingly high and remains inexplicable. Finally, as frequently noted, the young suffered unusually high mortality rates.

Cities only miles apart often had distinctly divergent experiences of the pandemic. Philadelphia, 100 miles southwest of Manhattan and NYC, experienced much different pandemics. The war had put both cities in a bind. NYC was the major embarkation point for troops headed to Europe and that wasn't going to stop. Philadelphia was a major naval base with ships and sailors constantly coming and going. New York City mobilised a massive multilingual public health effort and 'flattened the curve'. Philadelphia flouted public health advice and paid a deadly price with a fatality rate 50% higher than that of NYC.

NYC's Health Commissioner, Royal S. Copeland, a homeopathic optometrist, acted swiftly when he realised the extent of the epidemic. Although only on the job since April, in his favour was the department's 20 years of experience working to eradicate tuberculosis. Employers were ordered to introduce staggered work times to reduce rush hour crowding on public transit. Department literature was translated into Italian and Yiddish. Between vaudeville acts, department employees took to the stage to deliver public health lectures in all three languages. Interestingly Copeland closed neither public places of entertainment nor schools. His reasoning concerning the latter is instructive. He argued that classrooms were less crowded and cleaner than tenements and that students' health would suffer if they were not being fed at school. School was healthier than home for the poorest children in the city.

Philadelphia's response was too little, too late. In contrast to Copeland, Dr Wilmer Krusen, Director of Public Health and Charities for the city, insisted mounting fatalities were not due to the 'Spanish flu,' but rather just a severe seasonal flu. So on September 28, the city went forward with a Liberty Loan parade attended by tens of thousands of patriotic citizens. Ten days later more than 1000 Philadelphians were dead and another 200,000 sick. When the flu finally abated in the spring of 1919, more than 15,000 citizens of Philadelphia had lost their lives.

However, these were hardly the only cities affected. In Boston's Camp Devens, Dr Grist noted, "It is horrible... We have been averaging about 100 deaths per day." He also noted the ghastly consequences of this astronomical mortality rate, "For several days there were no coffins and the bodies piled up something fierce..." With the flu racing through the nursing staff, and the understaffed kitchen unable to provide meals, the Camp Devens base hospital stopped accepting patients.

In Goldsboro, North Carolina, Dan Tonkel recalled, "We were actually almost afraid to breathe... You were afraid even to go out... The fear was so great people were actually afraid to leave their homes... afraid to talk to one another." In Washington, D.C., William Sardo said, "It kept people apart... You had no school life, you had no church life, you had nothing... It completely destroyed all family and community life... The terrifying aspect was when each day dawned you didn't know whether you would be there when the sun set that day."

Such were the experiences of civilians. At the same time the flu was racing through the trenches from Flanders to the Argonne. In the context of a world war, one must consider its impact on the conflict. Specifically, was the combat effectiveness of any one army impaired significantly more or less than others?

On 3 August, 1918, before the Allied counter offensive started, Field-Marshal Rupprecht, Crown Prince of Bavaria noted wearily in his diary, "Poor provisions, heavy losses and the deepening influenza have deeply depressed the spirits of the men in the III Infantry Division." General Erich Ludendorff also took note that the loss of his men to influenza was undermining combat effectiveness. On the other hand, in late September, he told the army's Surgeon-General that the recent fresh outbreak of the pandemic in the French army might yet offer Germany a chance to negotiate their way out of the war. advantageously. The point being the disease seems to have affected all the armies relatively equally. According to Howard Phillips, University of Cape Town, "This ambiguous assertion is probably justified. Common sense dictates that the German army was not the only force affected by the pandemic." That said, while they were not the only army affected they may have been slightly more vulnerable than the Allied forces. By 1918 the British blockade was starving the German economy, as well as individual civilians and soldiers. During the German offensives in the spring of 1918 Prince Rupprecht complained that his offensives lost impetus because after a successful attack his troops refused to pursue the enemy until they had eaten and drunk any and all captured provisions. Malnourished, the Germans, soldiers and civilians alike, were probably more vulnerable than the other armies. Ernst Jünger saw this, "The sickness was also spreading among the enemy; even though we, with our poor rations, were more prone to it." Even if this were true by the fall of 1918 the armistice was only two months away and weightier factors had already doomed the Kaiser's armies.

While the pandemic had no impact on who won the war it may have had an impact on the peace. The armistice was followed by a gathering of world leaders at Versailles and while some were immune others were infected. British PM David Lloyd George had already had it earlier. President Woodrow Wilson was not as lucky and, arguably, he was the most important man at the conference. Despite minimal participation in combat the USA was emerging as a global power economically and strategically. Wilson's Fourteen Points were the unofficial agenda of the conference, but illness undermined him. It may have been more than just influenza, or the influenza may have led to strokes, but he returned from Europe seriously ill and neurologically impaired. Returning to the USA he was so enfeebled he was unable to persuade Congress to ratify the treaty. Consequently, the USA had no say as the signees sorted out the details, including reparations. Wilson had opposed a large indemnity, but the British and French imposed huge reparations which many see as a root cause of the Second World War.

The pandemic was unique in that it emerged during the dying days of a global war that had already killed an estimated 40 million over four years. It was a pandemic on the tail end of a global military catastrophe. Russia's war had ended in revolution and defeat. The French Army mutinied in 1917. For four years on the Western Front armies had lived below ground amid rats and lice, on a chemical soaked battleground that saw tanks, aircraft and machine-guns kill at an unprecedented pace. It so overwhelmed the public that it was known at the time as simply, 'the Great War', and later, with misplaced optimism, 'the War to End All Wars'.

These paired cataclysms make it almost impossible to tease out the consequences of the global war and separate them from the impact of the pandemic, or vice versa. Social and cultural historians concur that the 'Roaring Twenties' were typified by experimentation and extremism. Prohibition and bathtub gin, jazz and the Charleston, flappers and spiritualism were all aspects of the 1920s. However, to try to determine which arose from the war and which from the pandemic is often a mugs game; yet neither can they be denied. In the words of University of Cape Town historian Howard Phillips, "the Great War and the Great Flu were integral to each other in a host of interacting ways." The author of *Pale Rider*, Laura Spinney, concurs: "It isn't possible to disentangle the effects of flu and war on the psyche of those who were alive then, but perhaps it isn't necessary. The challenge is more modest: to demonstrate that the Spanish flu contributed to that psychological shift."

The remarkable rise of spiritualism provides a perfect illustration. As was the case with previous pandemics, in their aftermath they left an increased interest in religion and spirituality, specifically the fate and circumstances of the recently deceased. This was reflected in both a broader interest in spiritual activities and more extreme manifestations of religiosity. In the 1920s Spiritualism – the idea that the dead exist in a 'spirit world' and can be communicated with by the gifted – soared in popularity and ouija boards and seances became all the rage. The bizarre name, Ouija, has a perfectly logical origin. The inventor asked the board itself, and its ideo-motor effect or the afterworld, successively pointed out the letters, O-U-I-J-I (presumably the irregular plural of Ouija). It was so common that in May 1920, Norman Rockwell, iconic illustrator of American domesticity, depicted a man and a woman, Ouija board on their knees, communing with the beyond on the cover of the *Saturday Evening Post*.

Throughout the 1920s newspapers regularly reported amateur sleuths offering solutions to crimes and murders based on their erudite Ouija boards. Harry Houdini, an ardent opponent of all things spiritual and an active debunker, dismissed the Ouija board as, "the first step to insanity." The interest in spiritualism was pervasive, its origins are less clear. One cannot possibly separate the dead of the war from the dead of the flu, as inspiration.

The two most prominent proponents of spiritualism were British: Sir Arthur Conan Doyle and Sir Oliver Lodge. Doyle was, of course, the creator of Sherlock Holmes. Lodge was a respected physicist known for his work with radio waves. Both men had a longtime interest in the supernatural, and both had lost sons in the war. Lodge's son Raymond had been struck down by a shell fragment while fighting in Belgium in 1915. Doyle's son Kingsley had been wounded in France in 1916 and died of pneumonia in 1918, likely brought on by the influenza pandemic. Doyle also lost his younger brother to the flu in 1919, while his wife's brother had been killed in Belgium in 1914. Considering the dual die offs represented by the war and the influenza pandemic it is hardly surprising that interest in the dearly departed surfaced.

On the other hand, there are aftereffects of the influenza pandemic that can be directly linked to the pandemic. A plunge in life expectancy was clearly caused by the influenza pandemic. In just one year, 1918, the average life expectancy in America plummeted by a dozen years. This one year drop from 1917, a year that accounts for wartime casualties, to 1918 can be directly tied to the pandemic which eventually killed 675,000 Americans – almost 200,000 of whom died in one month, October, 1918. In Boston, 202 people died on just one day—October 1. Philadelphia later topped that record with 700 deaths in one 24-hour period. In Scandinavia, neutral, non-combatants, life expectancy fell from the mid-50s to the high 40s. This could only be a consequence of the pandemic as they experienced no combat fatalities.

Interestingly in light of the 2020 American Presidential election, the USA had to hold mid-term elections in November 1918, at the very peak of the pandemic. The result was accusations, countercharges and compromises. In New York, Democrat Alfred Smith was running to unseat Republican Governor Charles Whitman. In the *New York Times* he accused Republican officials of enacting bans in upstate cities to prevent him from campaigning: "A meeting had been scheduled for the City of Hornell on Monday night, Oct. 21, and in spite of the fact that there is little evidence of the epidemic in that city, as the schools, churches, and places of amusement are open... Of course, I have no intention of addressing meetings in localities where my doing so might involve a menace to the public health, but this idea of stopping meetings on the ground that the epidemic might strike a town by the time I get there as the Hornell authorities did, seems to me far fetched enough to justify suspicion that they want to prevent the spread of Democratic doctrine rather than the spread of Spanish influenza." Smith defeated Whitman by 13,000 votes.

The strangest case occurred in Cassia County Idaho. Nineteen teachers and students were quarantined on the Albion Normal School's 30 acre campus. Unable to leave quarantine, on Monday 4, November they appealed to the county commissioners requesting a precinct be established on the campus so they could exercise the franchise. Their request was granted and 19 ballots were cast. Democrat Frank Dotson won by four votes, but lost the recount by 11 votes to the Republican incumbent Thomas Harper. Dotson sued, arguing the 19 votes were cast illegally.

Clearly, the commissioners had violated the letter of the law, which plainly stated, "they must not alter or change any election precinct or change the place of holding election in any precinct after their regular July meeting next preceding any election". They had done so the day before the election, long after their July meeting. However, all three judges – a Republican and two Democrats – ruled that election laws were to be interpreted liberally if election officials acted in good faith and in response to local circumstances.

Nonetheless, the court disallowed the results for another reason. They argued that establishing precincts to accommodate quarantine was legal, provided the opportunity was announced publicly and offered widely. It was not, and as such constituted a 'special dispensation granted certain individuals' which betrayed the voting rights of everyone else in quarantine who had not had an equivalent opportunity. In light of the impending Presidential election in November 2020, the obscure Idaho case of Harper v. Dotson will be in the headlines again a century later. Unfortunately, it offers only ambiguous guidance at best.

Nationally, in fact, voter turnout fell from 50% in the 1914 mid-terms, to 40% in 1918. In the UK pre-1918 voter turnout figures are unavailable, however, for the 1918 election held in November, at the height of the pandemic, voter turnout was calculated at 57.1%, the lowest on record since. Four years later it had increased by a third to 73%. Recognising that voter turnout usually increases during wartime, this is a particularly significant shift. Despite the low turnout and irregularities the constitutionality of the election was never questioned.

On a broader scale though, the legitimacy of society, politics and the economy were being questioned. "Old authority and traditional values no longer had credibility... The 20s, as a result, witnessed a hedonism and narcissism of remarkable proportions... A profound sense of spiritual crisis was the hallmark of the decade," writes cultural historian Modris Eksteins.

The mayhem in the streets that terrorised residents of Chicago and New York City was only one of the most visible aspects of the hysteria that swept America during the 1920s. The decade began with the roundup of thousands of suspected 'Reds' and their fellow travellers. Unemployed veterans of the American Expeditionary Force, who had returned home as heroes in 1919, suddenly came to be viewed as a revolutionary threat to social stability. In January 1919, in the midst of the pandemic, the Seattle Central Labor Council (CLC) called a general strike and 35,000 workers, including all those at the shipyards and port, walked out; an ancestor to the establishment of the Capitol Hill Organized Protest (CHOP), demolished in late June, in Seattle during the COVID-19 pandemic.

In the fall of 1919, America's game was shattered by the revelations that the Chicago White Sox had thrown the World Series, (in what became known as the 'Black' Sox Scandal). Investigation of the scandal carried into the first years of the Twenties. Although baseball's popularity grew throughout the decade, it was never again the innocent pastime it had once been.

Fundamentalist preachers decried automobiles as 'bawdy houses on wheels' and Amiee Semple MacPherson preached from the vast Angelus Temple, the first megachurch, in California (until a staged kidnapping and rumours of assignations undermined her religiosity). In Kansas City, Reverend E. F. Stanton claimed that, "women who once dressed decently now wear clothes high and low. High at the bottom and low at the top." Jazz, increasingly popular, was decried as the devil's music and the Charleston was dismissed for its wonton sensuality. Diving horses and occasionally deadly dance marathons became all the rage. Automatic weapons and automobiles were the physical manifestations of the impact of the twin crises on American society. A sense of hysteria and existential crisis was a less visible, but more profound, impact.

On the other side of the fence, if slower to manifest, were the profound impacts on public health of the influenza pandemic. This was particularly true in New York, specifically its poorest and newest inhabitants: Italian immigrants. Dr Antonio Scalla, himself an Italian immigrant, was a respiratory specialist involved in the pandemic fight. In an effort to trace the disease he had students surveying the city's slums reporting the infected and incidentally recording conditions – persons per room, availability of water, a flush toilet, and so on. This project had two long term effects. Post pandemic this data revealed the horrible conditions in Manhattan tenements and forced municipal authorities to take action against landlords. It also led the city to initiate a public housing programme.

On the cultural level, Copeland's introduction of the compulsory hospitalisation of anyone registered ill with influenza smashed a psychological barrier. Many Italian immigrants had never seen a hospital let alone the inside of one and believed doctors were a luxury reserved for the rich. Mandatory hospitalisation introduced the unwilling to 'modern' medicine and weakened the stigma among the patients and their families. Thus, the pandemic introduced this group to modern medicine and improved their living conditions: One of the few benefits of this pandemic.

On a wider stage the overwhelming nature of the pandemic and its wide reach was a seminal event in the expansion of public health and public health care (as in socialised medicine) during the interwar years. Admittedly, this was an era of international organisations, typified by the League of Nations, but it is no coincidence that the International Committee of the Red Cross established a Vienna bureau under Dr Frédéric Ferrière dedicated to detecting and combating epidemics in 1919. In the same year in England, the Ministry of Health amalgamated the Local Government Board, the National Health Insurance Commissions for England and Wales and the Privy Council under the Midwives Acts, uniting all medical services under one government ministry. In the USA a national morbidity registry was established in 1925 and the Rockefeller Foundation became heavily involved in pandemic work. All of these developments reflected the twin realisations that public health was key to national productivity and security, and that pandemics could only be confronted by a united international front.

This pandemic can be said to have produced two very contradictory outcomes. On the one hand there was a psychological shift towards hysterical extremism evident in everything from radical politics of both the left and the right to gin and jazz. On the other hand, there was an increased awareness of public health and international organisation to confront pandemic infectious diseases.

The globe would survive another world war before another pandemic struck. However, since then, beginning with the influenza pandemic of 1957-58, the threat of zoonotic infectious pandemics has accelerated. The nature of the threats has changed and their frequency has increased. The risk of another global pandemic as unbelievably destructive as the 1918-1919 pandemic has increased every year for the past half century.

6.

The Pace Quickens

"Only behavior modification or medical management of this future health burden will minimise the risks of future zoonoses for human populations."

Michael G. Cordingley, President and Founder of
Revolution Pharma Consulting and Senior Scientific
Advisor at Antiva Biosciences

IN THE spring of 1919 the influenza pandemic slowly evaporated – leaving a confused and battered post-war world behind. But it was only a breather. The influenza pandemic widely known as Asian flu emerged in 1957-1958. A new influenza A (H2N2) virus emerged in East Asia after zoonosis from an avian virus. It was first reported in Singapore in February 1957, Hong Kong two months later, and in coastal cities in the United States that summer. Case fatality rates were about 0.67%. The estimated number of deaths was 1.1 million worldwide, 116,000 in the United States and 33,000 in the UK.

Just a decade later, the 1968 Hong Kong flu pandemic, subtype H3N2, emerged in China and spread throughout Europe and North America, reaching Australia by early 1969. Although mortality rates were relatively low, the pandemic would ultimately claim between 500,000 and two million lives. Edwin D. Kilbourne notes also three other influenza pandemics that were narrowly dodged: "Not classified as true pandemics are three notable epidemics: a pseudopandemic in 1947 with low death rates, an epidemic in 1977 that was a pandemic in children, and an abortive epidemic of swine influenza in 1976 that was feared to have pandemic potential."

H1N1 emerged again in the swine flu epidemic of 2009. It was a bizarre subtype that combined human, avian and swine RNA. It is such a confusing recombinant that a decade later its origin remains unknown. A Mexican factory farm and several small farms in central Mexico and China have all been suggested. What is known is it was first detected in Mexico and California in March 2009. Mexico City was locked down. In June the WHO and CDC declared it a pandemic. In 2012 the CDC Influenza Division estimated a range of deaths between 150,000 and 575,000 during the first year the virus circulated with more than half of all deaths occurring in Southeast Asia and Africa.

This brief summary hides terrifying news. In the five decades following the 1957-58 influenza pandemic there have been two other influenza pandemics and three near misses, every one the product of recombinant zoonosis. The pace quickens and the plot thickens because zoonotic influenza pandemics are only the tip of the iceberg. In *Epidemics and Society* Frank Snowden enumerates recent zoonotic infections: "The list includes HIV, Hantavirus, Lassa fever, Marburg fever, Legionnaires' disease, hepatitis C, Lyme disease, Rift Valley fever, Ebola, Nipah virus, West Nile virus, SARS, bovine spongiform encephalopathy, avian flu, Chikungunya virus, norovirus, Zika, and group A streptococcus—the so-called flesh-eating bacterium." The WHO documented 1100 epidemic events between 2002 and 2007. A brief summary of some of these other pandemics will demonstrate that the pace is reaching warp speed.

Looking back 40 years, HIV is a zoonotic virus. It passed from chimpanzees to humans, probably in the 1920s. Chimps are carnivores and often eat smaller primates. These prey were infected with two strains of Simian Immunodeficiency Virus (SIV). Recombinant drift within the chimps gave rise to a third strain (SIVcpz), a virus that could also infect humans. The resultant virus mutated within humans enabling human-to-human transmission and the outcome was the AIDS pandemic.

Looking towards COVID-19, there is one unavoidable lesson from the HIV/AIDS pandemic. While there are a wide range of therapeutics and treatments for AIDS and it is now viewed as a chronic condition rather than a death sentence, there is no vaccine. Politicians were promising a vaccine for COVID-19 within 40 days when in other cases there has been no vaccine within 40 years. The mumps vaccine, developed faster than any other vaccine, required four years. Four decades on, HIV/AIDS remains a lived experience. For this reason 'life after COVID-19' does not refer to life after the disease is *eliminated* but rather, life after the disease was *introduced*.

Ebola

The Ebola virus (EBOV) was first discovered in 1976 near the Ebola River in what is now the Democratic Republic of Congo (thought to be the region of origin for HIV as well). The natural wildlife host of EBOV has not been definitively identified but evidence suggests fruit bats of the family *Pteropodidae* might be a reservoir. Bats are thought to play a role in transmission of COVID-19 also. The index patient (the first case) of the Ebola pandemic was reported in December 2013 and it soon spread to Guinea's capital city of Conakry. On August 8, 2014, the WHO declared the deteriorating situation in West Africa a Public Health Emergency of International Concern (PHEIC) which is designated only for events with a risk of potential international spread or that require a coordinated international response. Concurrently there was another outbreak in the Democratic Republic of Congo (DRC). Ebola remains endemic in Africa.

Ebola spillover most commonly occurs in two manners: blood from hunting and butchering bush meat can enter the body through a cut; eating undercooked or uncooked bush meat is the second avenue of infection. Subsequent transmission to family members often occurs when burying the dead. The Ebola virus remains infectious long after death – so if family members prepare the body traditionally by themselves the risk of infection is phenomenally high. Changes in behaviours related to mourning and burial, along with the adoption of safe burial practices, were critical in controlling Ebola.

No UK residents have died from Ebola and the only American to die was a nurse infected while doing humanitarian work in Africa. As one headline writer put it, "More Americans Have Been Married to Kim Kardashian than Have Died of Ebola". But Ebola inspired a global panic. Travel bans, quarantine of all returnees from Africa and all measure of extreme reactions occurred. Social media coined the term Ebolanoia. In the USA, anti-immigration hawks accused illegal immigrants of bringing it over the borders of the USA and the CDC had to assure the nation that it was impossible to get Ebola from an undercooked Thanksgiving turkey.

Science journalist Sonia Shaw documents the most extreme overreach: "A school board in Maine went so far as to compel a teacher to quarantine herself after she attended a conference in Dallas because it was held ten miles away from a hospital where a man who'd been infected with Ebola in Liberia had been treated." It was an Orson Welles 'War of the Worlds' fit of hysteria that ultimately amounted to much ado about nothing outside of specific regions in Africa. That said, it is not uncommon for pandemics to foster hysteria although the extremity of this case is atypical.

Of note is the world's response to this outbreak. A global effort saw international health workers pouring into the affected areas. UN Mission for Ebola Emergency Response (UNMEER), the first-ever UN emergency health mission, was established on September 19, 2014, and closed on July 31, 2015, having achieved its core objective of scaling up the response on the ground. On that date the medical mission was handed off to the WHO. The coordinated, rapid global response managed to control community spread and limit infections and fatalities.

Zika

Zika Virus Disease (ZVD) is a mosquito-borne flavivirus that was first identified in Uganda in 1947 in monkeys. It was later identified in humans in 1952 in Uganda and the United Republic of Tanzania. Like Yellow Fever, Zika is spread mostly by the bite of an infected *Aedes* species mosquito (*Ae. aegypti* and *Ae. albopictus*) the same mosquitos that killed off Napoleon's expeditionary force. The virus replicates in the human testis and transmission is primarily sexual. Zika presents particular risks to pregnant women as it has been linked to birth defects, specifically microcephaly.

This brief survey of pandemics since 1918 illustrates the increasing rate at which zoonotic infections are emerging. Snowden's dire warning, "The number of previously unknown conditions that have emerged to afflict humanity since 1970 exceeds 40, with a new disease discovered on average more than once a year," is hardly encouraging. Most importantly, every time a zoonotic infection spills over from an animal reservoir we (*homo sapiens*) are all a virgin population with absolutely no immunity. And, on that pessimistic note, it is time to meet the pathogens currently bedevilling us.

SARS

First identified in 2003 after several months of cases, Severe Acute Respiratory Syndrome (SARS) is another zoonotic disease believed to have possibly started with bats, spread to cats and then to humans, in China. SARS is characterised by respiratory problems, dry cough, fever and head and body aches and is spread through respiratory droplets from coughs and sneezes. It is a coronavirus, an introduction to the family of viruses that includes COVID-19.

Coronaviruses consist of a ball containing the virus's RNA wreathed (Latin-*corona*) with protein spikes. Their discoverers wrote, "We looked more closely at the appearance of the new viruses and noticed that they had a kind of halo surrounding them." The halo is composed of E, M and S proteins. The large red S proteins are key to infection. They adhere to the 'victim' cell and like a microbial mosquito they 'bite' the host cell, allowing the virus to insert its RNA. The viral RNA then hijacks the host cell's DNA and the host cell, rather than reproducing itself, begins reproducing the virus. As the viral load increases the host sickens and, possibly, dies.

With zoonotic viruses the human immune system is powerless. The question becomes, how infectious is the virus? A zoonotic disease that passes from an animal reservoir to a human may initially be transmissible also directly from human to human. If it is not it needs to mutate until that ability emerges. Unfortunately, since viruses only contain RNA and must borrow DNA they can mutate with startling rapidity. In a Darwinian process, mutations that permit human to human transmission proliferate and come to predominate. The result is a pandemic.

Toronto, the capital of Canada's most populous province was slammed by SARS. It was the only city outside of Asia to suffer SARS deaths. Its arrival in Toronto speaks to the astronomical pace at which a pandemic can span the globe. A Hong Kong couple's wedding was attended by a doctor from Guangdong who was asymptomatic but infected. A woman from Toronto also attended and brought the virus home with her. The virus covered half of the globe in a matter of days. It also explains, in this modern era of air travel, how outbreaks can occur in widely separated locations but be directly connected. The 19th century concern with disease travelling at the speed of steamships and railroads hardly compares.

The woman infected her family before she died at home. Scarborough Hospital, where the woman's son died, had to be closed. The provincial government declared a health emergency on March 23, 2003, and 'Code Orange' emergency plans were activated. Hospitals were closed to visitors and elective surgeries were cancelled. In mid-April, the WHO issued a travel advisory that included Toronto, the only city outside of Asia. Eventually, the outbreak was contained with only 44 deaths, largely because SARS was only mildly infectious. Between hospital closures, quarantines and other restrictions it is estimated that the disease caused Toronto's GDP to take a hit to the tune of $1 billion. Overall, national healthcare costs were estimated at $2 billion.

In the aftermath of the outbreak, governments at all levels produced reports, commissions and investigations. The Public Health Agency of Canada (PHAC) produced *Learning from SARS*, concluding that Canada was ill-prepared for a pandemic: "Enhancement of surveillance mechanisms, better coordination among the various levels of government and institutions for outbreak containment, improved public communications strategies, and major increases in expert human resources are just some of the changes needed if Canada is to be better prepared for future health crises."

COVID-19 is challenging these public health systems again and 18 years on there is still no vaccine for SARS.

MERS

A decade after SARS a second zoonotic coronavirus emerged. Middle East Respiratory Syndrome (MERS) is a viral respiratory illness caused by MERS-CoV. According to the WHO, "dromedary camels are a major reservoir host for MERS-CoV and an animal source of MERS infection in humans. However, the exact role of dromedaries in transmission of the virus and the exact route(s) of transmission are unknown."

Its symptoms are typical of severe respiratory illness; fever, cough and shortness of breath. The CFR is very high, estimated at 30-40%. However, human to human transmission is rare, seemingly limited to close contact (i.e. healthcare workers). Health officials first reported the disease in Saudi Arabia in September 2012 and subsequently 'Patient Zero' was traced to Jordan the previous spring. "Most infected people either lived in the Arabian Peninsula or recently travelled from the Arabian Peninsula before they became ill", the CDC reported at the time. The largest known outbreak of MERS outside the Arabian Peninsula occurred in the Republic of Korea in 2015 and caused 38 deaths. The virus was imported by a traveller returning from the Arabian Peninsula, with ensuing hospital-to-hospital transmission. Again, eight years later there is no vaccine for MERS.

COVID-19

And so, two zoonotic coronavirus pandemics this century bring the story to the present. They follow a century teeming with pandemics and they set the stage for the present pandemic and future life after COVID-19. At the time of writing, during the fall of 2020 and with the pandemic raging, it is impossible to avoid questions about preparedness or lack thereof, specifically the underfunding of public health. A post mortem or detailed analysis of the particular failures of any one national government is beyond the scope of this book. Suffice to say that no government can claim to have been adequately prepared for a pandemic and a handful of points will illustrate this.

Under the headline, "Why We're Losing the Battle With COVID-19", in *The New York Times Magazine*, Jeneen Interlandi argued, "the chronic under-funding of public health has put America on track for the worst coronavirus response in the developed world". The stark facts she presents to support her case are shocking. "Health departments across the country have seen their budgets shrink by nearly 30% since 2008. As a result, they have had to cut 56,000 jobs (nearly 23% of the total public-health work force)." Capital purchases of laboratory equipment and computer systems have been cancelled or deferred. Nationally the CDC budget has not increased in a decade, programmes directed at infectious disease have shrunk and data collection methods are incomplete and archaic.

In England, *The British Medical Journal* was as blunt as the NYT. An editorial entitled, "How the erosion of our public health system hobbled England's COVID-19 response" details "savage cuts" to public health with the inevitable consequences. Pre-pandemic public health budgets were out of sight and out of mind.

Canada, specifically Toronto, having dodged a SARS bullet, should have been more prepared than most for a pandemic. It had been. After SARS, Canada stockpiled PPE. However, with a five-year shelf life it was (incredibly) disposed of in 2008. After the H1N1 outbreak in 2009, Canada stockpiled again. And in May 2019 the federal government landfilled two million expired N95 masks, and did not replace them. Dr Andrew Morris, an infectious disease specialist at Toronto's Sinai Health and University Health Network, argued there was no excuse for this failure, "I think a lot of this relates to the chronic underfunding of public health in Ontario. Many of the problems that we're experiencing today were experienced during [the 2002-2003] SARS crisis as well... Our public health infrastructure has really not ramped up to the level that we've needed to." SARS was an early warning sign for Toronto and Canada, yet neither were prepared for COVID-19. Failing to buy a spare tyre saves money but COVID-19 is the flat in the middle of nowhere in the middle of the night when its raining.

Data collection has been an issue in Canada too. Amir Attaran, a professor in the Faculty of Law and the School of Epidemiology and Public Health at the University of Ottawa, uses a particularly Canadian analogy to illuminate the data problems, "I cannot exaggerate how dangerous such blindness is. Without complete, accurate, timely data Canada fights COVID-19 not by skating to where the virus's puck is going, or even where it is now, but where it was several weeks ago." What we know is that the 'puck' today is a global pandemic of inconceivable scale.

Officially, the virus has been christened SARS-CoV-2 and the disease, COVID-19. Some tall tales have been bandied around since the outbreak commenced: It is not a product of the National Bio-safety Laboratory in Wuhan as some American sources have suggested. Neither was it brought to Wuhan by the US military for the Military World Games in October 2019.

A mundane explanation of its origins is more than adequate. It is simply the most recent case of zoonosis. The process of a virus making the leap from animals to humans has happened with increasing frequency in the recent past and it was inevitable it would happen again. As Dr Anthony Fauci explained to National Geographic in May 2020: "If you look at the evolution of the virus in bats, and what's out there now is very, very strongly leaning toward this [virus] could not have been artificially or deliberately manipulated – the way the mutations have naturally evolved. A number of very qualified evolutionary biologists have said that everything about the stepwise evolution over time strongly indicates that it evolved in nature and then jumped species." It spilled over and mutated to enable human-to-human transmission. It is the pandemic that has been dodged for the last century.

Setting aside the official designation, the virus has had, as President Trump noted, 19 different names. Frequently, it is referred to as the 'novel' coronavirus and that is the root of our current problem. Novel means more than merely new, it implies novelty and uniqueness, and that is what makes SARS-CoV-2 so dangerous. The entire human species is a virgin population. Human immune systems have never encountered this pathogen before and have no resistance. For this reason also, doctors and scientists are dealing with an immense unknown. As Dr Gregory Poland, director of the Mayo Clinic vaccine research group, confessed in June, "everything we know about this virus is what, 22, 23 weeks old." Implicit in this admission is recognition of the fact that there are currently neither a vaccine to prevent COVID-19 nor therapeutics to treat it. Non-pharmaceutical interventions are the only tools in the tool box. That is why, as noted earlier, 'social distancing is the only vaccine we have to fight this deadly virus' in the fall of 2020.

In Germany, Sunday, November 17, 2019 (the second Sunday in the church year) was Volkstrauertag (The National Day of Mourning) a Stillertag (Silent Day) established in the 1920s to recognise the dead of the recent war and pandemic. On that same Sunday a 55-year-old man in Hubei province sought medical help with flu-like symptoms. Life before COVID-19 was over.

Five months later, at the time of writing in the fall of 2020, the disease is present in 213 countries. There have been 25 million confirmed cases of COVID-19 (a number which in no way is an accurate measure as it only includes persons tested). Of these 6.6 million are ill at present and 16.4 million people have recovered. Approximately 830,000 individuals have died, producing a case fatality rate (CFR) globally of 5%. The USA has conducted more tests than any other country as President Trump has often boasted. However, it also leads in terms of total cases and total deaths, with a CFR of 5%. The almost six million cases in the USA puts it way out in front of the next three countries – Brazil (3.6m cases), India (3.1m cases) and Russia (0.9m cases).

The UK has had only 330,000 cases but it has a frighteningly high CFR of 12.7% leaving more than 40,000 dead. A handful of countries have reported no cases, primarily small island nations such as the Marshall Islands, Micronesia, Nauru, Palau and Samoa. North Korea and Turkmenistan also report being virus free although the veracity of their reports is questionable. Briefly, this is how a pandemic emerges. Twenty-five million infections in a little over eight months, and the number is growing. More than 800,000 dead. All of these trends are accelerating. Some suggest this is a second wave a la 1918, others claim the first wave is not over yet. What is clear is the pandemic shows no signs of abating.

It has even worked its way into the lifestyles of the rich and famous. Most notably, British PM Boris Johnson had to be hospitalised himself after shaking hands with COVID-19 patients and Tom Hanks' diagnosis made the Hollywood headlines. Prince Charles too was infected but quickly recovered and children's author Michael Rosen spent nearly seven weeks in intensive care, much of that time in a medically induced coma, before pulling through. In Canada, Sophie Grégoire Trudeau was infected and forced to self-isolate along with her husband, Canadian Prime Minister Justin Trudeau. Katie Miller, Vice-President Mike Pence's press secretary (and wife of close Trump aide Stephen Miller) was infected, as were National Security Adviser Robert O'Brien and Oklahoma Governor Kevin Stitt. For some it has proven fatal, including actor Nick Cordero, musicians John Prine, Adam Schlesinger, Dave Greenfield and Ellis Marsalis Jr., artist Paul Karslake, and comics Eddie Large and Tim Brooke-Taylor. The list goes on and on.

Elsewhere, and not surprisingly, a pandemic is a very bad time to be inside a prison. Prior to his pardon by President Trump, political operative Roger Stone's lawyer argued that the threat of the virus should delay his reporting to prison. It did not work, although a Presidential pardon allowed him to escape incarceration. It was a legitimate concern. Overcrowding, poor sanitation, limited personal hygiene facilities, communal transportation, work and dining all make prisons an ideal environment for the virus.

In England, *The Guardian* has referred to the situation as a crisis. In April the UK government authorised the release of up to 5200 prisoners to reduce overcrowding. But as of July 1 only 175 had been granted early release. According to the Ministry of Justice, 510 inmates had been infected and 23 have died (to July 1, 2020). However, *The Guardian* alleged testing had been inadequate and the Ministry refused to release detailed figures. Its statistics indicate the number of cases per million is 50% higher in prison than among the wider population.

In Canada, the public broadcaster documented similar problems: "A preliminary analysis by CBC News suggests that, despite prevention measures such as releasing thousands of low-risk offenders, infection rates are still five times higher in provincial jails and up to nine times higher in federal facilities than in the general population."

In the USA JAMA reported, in the second week of July, that COVID-19 cases in US federal and state prisons were 5.5 times higher than in the general population between March 31 and June 6. Over the same period the death rate was triple that of the general population. These aggregate figures bury some terrifying specifics; "Mass testing in select prisons revealed wide COVID-19 outbreaks, with infection rates exceeding 65% in several facilities." These North American statistics make the UK's Ministry of Justice estimate of a rate 0.5 times higher than the general population seem as unbelievable as *The Guardian* has suggested. Prisons are designed to warehouse criminals at minimal expense and it is not surprising that they are crowded, dirty and dangerous during a pandemic.

The same cannot be said of the elderly. The Office for National Statistics (ONS) reported 16,000 deaths of seniors from COVID-19 to June 5, 2020 in England and Wales, more than one-third of total COVID-19 deaths. Comparatively, those figures are terrible, "The proportion of residents dying in UK homes was a third higher than in Ireland and Italy, about double that in France and Sweden, and 13 times higher than Germany," according to the ONS. Of all the UK's care home residents, 5.3% were confirmed or suspected to have died from COVID-19, compared with 0.4% in Germany, according to analysis of official statistics. In the USA four out of five COVID-19 fatalities were senior citizens.

The National Institute on Aging (Canada) reported in mid-May that 82% of all COVID-19 casualties were residents of long term care homes (LTCs). The Canadian Institute for Health Information published *Pandemic Experience in the Long-Term Care Sector: How Does Canada Compare With Other Countries?* in June 2020. It reported, "Canada's long-term care (LTC) sector has been especially hard hit by the COVID-19 pandemic. More than 840 outbreaks have been reported in LTC facilities and retirement homes, accounting for more than 80% of all COVID-19 deaths in the country." The situation was extremely dire in the Canadian province of Ontario where Premier Rob Ford had to ask the federal government to send in Canadian military medical personnel and hospitals assembled emergency medical teams to move into LTCs, taking over patient care and sanitation.

That decision will have profound consequences in Ontario, and to a lesser extent Quebec – a second province that requested military assistance.

The military personnel were appalled by the conditions they encountered and issued scathing, public reports on both provinces' LTCs. Brief excerpts follow: "nearly a dozen incidents of bleeding fungal infections … Expired medication. Residents have likely been getting expired medication for quite some time... Insect infestation noted within LTC – ants and cockroaches plus unknown observed… Forceful feeding observed by staff causing audible choking/aspiration, forceful hydration causing audible choking/aspiration." Enough said.

The horrible conditions of malnutrition and dehydration made the elderly residents even more vulnerable. While the pandemic did not cause these problems – decades of cutbacks and privatisation under governments of all political stripes did that – it brought them to light (or brought in the military who finally made this dirty little secret public property). The sequelae of this episode will not fade away and with similar shocking statistics (if not revelations) in England and the USA, LTCs and nursing homes are bound to see significant changes.

Prisoners and nursing home residents are institutionalised and that structural factor goes a long way to explaining their elevated rates of infection.

The same cannot be said of other demographic groups that exhibit elevated levels of infection and mortality including Black, Asian, and Minority Ethnic (BAME) communities. Public Health England released *Beyond the Data: Understanding the Impact of COVID-19 on BAME Groups* in mid-June. Its conclusions were stark, "people of Bangladeshi ethnicity had around twice the risk of death when compared to people of White British ethnicity. People of Chinese, Indian, Pakistani, Other Asian, Caribbean and Other Black ethnicity had between 10 and 50% higher risk of death when compared to White British." On July 19, *The Guardian* reported that minority ethnic patients comprised 34% of critically ill COVID-19 patients in the UK despite constituting only 14% of the population.

In North America, on both sides of the border, a similar pattern has emerged. The CDC reported in the last week of June that whites had the lowest rate of hospitalisation among all ethnic groups in the USA. American Indian, Alaska Native persons and non-Hispanic black persons have a rate of hospitalisation of approximately five times that of non-Hispanic white persons, while Hispanic or Latino persons have a rate approximately four times that of non-Hispanic white persons.

In Canada, Public Health Ontario reported in June that neighbourhoods with the highest concentrations of new immigrants and ethnic minorities were four times higher, and death rates were twice as high as those in the least diverse neighbourhoods.

In New York City the Hispanic community had higher rates of infection and mortality than blacks. However, this ran against a national trend that saw black communities savaged. In late May as the United States passed 100,000 COVID-19 fatalities MSNBC reported that African Americans comprised 13% of the US population, yet they accounted for 23% of COVID-19 fatalities. The report traced the high rate to three underlying factors. African Americans are more likely to have underlying conditions such as diabetes, hypertension and asthma. Income inequalities and inadequate housing also contribute. Finally, the USA's patchwork, private health insurance system limits access to the healthcare system. Poverty and ethnicity are intertwined in American history and the present pandemic.

A century ago, doctors dealing with the influenza pandemic had never seen a virus and thought they were contending with a bacterial infection.

That is certainly no longer the case. Today doctors can produce images of the virus with electron microscopes and knew its genetic sequence within weeks of first encountering it. Doctors, however, have virtually no pharmaceutical interventions. At the time of writing, there is no vaccine and there are very few therapeutics and they are of limited utility.

Unlike doctors a century ago, medical researchers and epidemiologists are currently pouring money and resources into addressing COVID-19. Potential vaccines are moving into Stage 3 trials and hundreds of therapeutic possibilities are being explored. The scientific effort exceeds even the 'all hands on deck' effort the USA made in the 1960s to put a man on the moon. Governments, corporations, universities and hospitals are exploring a host of options and alternatives.

An old school treatment that made a brief appearance during the influenza pandemic, convalescent plasma, is being reconsidered. The first Nobel Prize awarded in Physiology and Medicine (1901) went to Emil von Behring, the 'Saviour of Children'. He developed a diphtheria antitoxin from antibodies taken from animals that had recovered from the disease. It made an appearance during the influenza pandemic and during the depression Dr J Roswell managed to stave off a measles outbreak at a boys' school in Pennsylvania by injecting the students with blood serum from a classmate who had survived the disease.

"Convalescent plasma has been used throughout history when confronting an infectious disease where you have people who recover and there's no other therapy available," says Warner Greene, director of the Centre for HIV Cure Research at the Gladstone Institutes. He concludes, "Convalescent plasma is the crudest of immunotherapies, but it can be effective." JAMA reports, "Studies are under way to evaluate use of convalescent plasma as treatment for patients with severe COVID-19 and to prevent infection (prophylaxis) in certain high-risk patients exposed to COVID-19. Convalescent plasma might provide immunity by giving patients neutralising antibodies for SARS-CoV-2."

Another old school method involves repurposing existing drugs. The list of possible drugs to repurpose includes lopinavir/ritonavir, favipiravir, tocilzumab and, notably, remdesivir. In May 2020, the National Institute of Allergy and Infectious Diseases (NIAID) led by Dr Anthony Fauci reported remdesivir was associated with a 31% quicker recovery time based on length of hospital stay. Subsequent studies have corroborated these results suggesting hospital stays are reduced on average from 15 days to 11 days. Remdesivir does not reduce mortality however. Sick people who survive get better more quickly, that is all. Remdesivir is a huge step forward but it is neither a cure nor a preventative.

With COVID-19 being a respiratory infection, nebulizers and inhalers are also being investigated as drug delivery systems. Experiments with existing aerosol steroids have demonstrated some success in relieving symptoms, but the most promising treatment is protein based. On July 20, the BBC reported, "The findings suggest the treatment cut the odds of a COVID-19 patient in hospital developing severe disease – such as requiring ventilation – by 79%... [and] the average time patients spent in hospital is said to be reduced by a third, for those receiving the new drug – down from an average of nine to six days."

Again, this is neither a preventative nor a cure. However, the reduction in the number of patients being intubated is significant. Intubation is incredibly intrusive and time spent in a medically induced coma is dangerous and damaging. Intubated patients who survive COVID-19 have a very poor prognosis, so any treatment that reduces the need for assisted breathing is a big step forward.

Regeneron, the American pharmaceutical giant, announced the initiation of Phase 3 late-stage clinical trials evaluating REGN-COV2, Regeneron's investigational double antibody cocktail for the treatment and prevention of COVID-19 on July 6. The drug is a combination of the strongest antibodies from two sources – recovered patients and mice genetically modified to have near-human immune systems. It is being investigated as both a preventative and a treatment and shows considerable promise.

The holy grail for medical researchers, the objective of the bizarrely named 'Operation Warp Speed', is a vaccine. Three candidates moving into Phase 3 in August 2020 clearly lead the field. On July 15, Moderna in partnership with 'Operation Warp Speed', announced Phase 3 trials on its RNA-platform vaccine would commence in two weeks. The Chinese company, CanSinoBIO was initiating Phase 3 trials on a potential vaccine based on an inactivated virus. In England, *The Lancet* reported on July 20 that an Oxford University/AstraZeneca collaboration, the ChAdOx1nCoV-19 vaccine (commonly referred to as AZD 1222), in a single-blind, randomised controlled trial had significant success. It relies on a non-replicating viral vector. Importantly, it triggered a dual response, increasing both antibodies and T-cells: Antibodies kill viruses, T-cells kill infected cells. In a vaccine this is ideal, and AZD 1222 is the most promising of the vaccine candidates. Both Russia and North Korea assert they have vaccines although these claims are widely dismissed.

The news on the vaccine front is encouraging but Phase 3 trials are only the beginning. The first version of the mumps vaccine developed in four years only provided short-term immunity. Jonas Salk spent eight years developing the polio vaccine. Dr Anthony Fauci has dedicated most of his career to HIV/AIDS research but 40 years on a vaccine remains unattainable. A vaccine will definitely not be a quick thing and it is not even a sure thing. Former CDC director Julie Geberding summed it up for CNN, "I think the science is on our side. That doesn't say anything about the speed, the safety and the durability and all of the other criteria that have to come into play before we have something that we can count on to give us that population immunity." That the first vaccine will be developed in weeks, that it will have a spectacular success rate and that it will endure is a pipe dream.

The issue of durability is particularly important with regard to COVID-19. Research indicates that immunity to COVID-19 is transient; simply put, the immune system forgets and immunity wears off. This being the case, one could get COVID-19, recover and a year later get it again because the immunity had faded. There is every reason to believe that the same transitory immunity will follow from a vaccination.

Any successful vaccine would raise a whole series of new issues. Rushed to market, the question of a new vaccine's long term safety would linger. The first vaccine might only work for certain demographics. Industry would have to gear up to produce millions of doses. Only then would the touchiest problem emerge: how would a vaccine be distributed? Could the wealthy purchase a private stock? Could Elon Musk buy enough for himself and key employees at Tesla? Would frontline workers get priority or would politicians and professional athletes have pride of place? Would President Trump hoard it to 'Make America Great Again'? Production and distribution of the first vaccines will be a highly contentious issue.

Once an effective vaccine is available, Joshua M. Epstein of the NYU School of Global Health worries that it will confront anti-vaxxer sentiments and campaigns. A vaccine is useless if it is not taken and herd immunity is predicated on a 90% plus vaccination rate. He notes, "Fear-driven vaccine refusal is responsible for the resurgence of measles in the US and Europe and even polio in many countries. We cannot rule out the possibility that vaccine refusal will undermine the worldwide effort to bring this new coronavirus to heel." He pessimistically concludes, "A third contagion, fear of the vaccine, could push us over the threshold into a renewed epidemic." Anti-vax misinformation will be amplified by the newness of the vaccine and the haste with which it was developed.

The issue of vaccines has another unexpected, but understandable, downside. During the pandemic children have been missing their regular vaccinations. Parents may be avoiding crowded doctors' offices while children who relied on school vaccination programmes have been locked out. A CDC study found a 'notable' year-over-year drop in orders for measles vaccines and other non-influenza childhood vaccines. "Between March 13 and April 19, doctors ordered 2.5 million fewer doses of non-influenza vaccines and 250,000 fewer doses of measles vaccines compared to last year", according to Politico. The terrifying fact is that one consequence of COVID-19 may be a resurgence in totally unrelated infectious and potentially pandemic childhood diseases.

Above and beyond the immediacy of finding a pharmaceutical intervention for COVID-19, Fauci has floated a novel idea that merits a long, long-term look. Fauci has argued that a 'platform' vaccine needs to be developed. This platform could then be tweaked to deal with variant coronaviruses. It is similar to the way the seasonal flu vaccine is tweaked each year, but on a much greater scale. Fauci rightly argues that if this had been done in the wake of SARS-CoV in 2003 we would be much better prepared for SARS-CoV-2 today. Ideally, research in this direction will be one of the beneficial impacts of COVID-19.

Toronto had a close brush with a pandemic and still did not learn its lesson. It was not alone; pandemic planning and preparedness was painfully inadequate across the map. This is hardly surprising as it is nothing new. Recall, Daniel Defoe crying in the wilderness while the plague ravaged Marseilles. In Halifax, Nova Scotia, no preparations were made for the 1834 visitation of cholera because a small fortune had been spent two years earlier on an epidemic that never happened. Pandemic disease planners face an eternal dilemma: if nothing happens they wasted money, if a pandemic erupts they didn't do enough. They are forced to ask politicians operating with a four-year horizon to prepare for a once-in-a-century event. Not surprisingly, most politicians decide it won't happen on their watch.

Historians and geographers, doctors and medical researchers, national security specialists and bureaucrats all warned of a future pandemic. The last 40 years, from HIV/AIDS to COVID-19, saw a host of 'warning signals' given and many opportunities for taking precautions were missed. The past can provide lessons for the present and the future. The repeated bubonic plagues were a warning, the influenza pandemic a century ago was a warning. This century SARS and MERS called us out and still COVID-19 caught us with our pants down. SARS-CoV-2 is here to stay for the foreseeable future and the only option, for now, is learning to live with it.

7.

Life After COVID-19

"People ask me if I'm worried and I say that you would have to be a fool to not be worried. The problem isn't just that there's no playbook for this. It's that nobody is even calling any plays."

Mayor Dan Gelber, Miami Beach, FL

VARIOUS LEVELS of government have offered guidance on non-pharmaceutical interventions to control the spread of COVID-19 that cover common ground – face coverings, social distancing, limiting interactions and handwashing. The mayor of Oakland, California, Libby Schaaf's pithy turn of phrase, "Social distancing is the only vaccine we have to fight this deadly virus", has proven painfully true. However, these measures to control the spread or flatten the curve are trivial compared to the more fundamental revolutionary changes occurring. COVID-19's overwhelming sequelae will fundamentally and forever alter our world in every sense; economically and politically, socially and culturally. It is not hyperbole to assert that COVID-19 will have the greatest impact of any pandemic event since the Black Death. Nor is it a stretch to assert that past pandemics offer valuable lessons on life after COVID-19.

COVID-19 will have an enduring physical effect on survivors along with mental health consequences for large swathes of the population. Gregory Poland, professor of medicine and infectious diseases at The Mayo Clinic, and director of the Mayo vaccine research group, raised two important questions, "Does it do other things to the brain? And there's been some initial suggestions that yes, it does. What about long term effects on a fetus? No one knows yet." Rany Condos, director of the advanced lung disease programme at NYU Langone Health, shared these concerns, "The lung is not the only organ that was involved in this pandemic. Many of the patients have had neurologic abnormalities. A lot of them have kidney abnormalities. We're going to see that there is a significant healthcare burden that's going to be associated with the COVID pandemic for a very long time." He also sees mental health costs in the future. "A lot of them [COVID-19 patients] are having symptoms of post traumatic stress. Some of them have anxiety. Some of them are showing signs of depression."

These mental health effects on families of survivors, on people unable to cope with lockdown and on children have been widely noted. In the early stages of the lockdown, the WHO issued a statement that warned of "elevated rates of stress or anxiety" in the general population, before stating that, "as new measures and impacts are introduced – especially quarantine and its effects on many people's usual activities, routines or livelihoods – levels of loneliness, depression, harmful alcohol and drug use, and self-harm or suicidal behaviour are also expected to rise."

Mike Davis, author of *The Monster at Our Door: The Global Threat of Avian Flu*, tweeted on March 16, "Indeed the combined effects of fear, confinement, income loss and the potential destruction of family savings augur a mental health crisis on an even larger scale than the pandemic itself. This isn't simply collateral damage but rather an integral and extremely dangerous part of the health threat that has so far been neglected." Psychotherapist Susie Orbach equated it with war or displacement, "The pandemic has been a prolonged assault from outside on our community. The state of uncertainty and unsafety it has created is new and utterly unfamiliar... There is simply nothing to compare it to." The physical and mental health consequences of COVID-19 will reverberate for at least a generation.

Jobs and the workplace

Social distancing and electronically mediated communication look set to become the norm, the default setting. According to Deborah Tannen, a professor of linguistics at Georgetown, "The comfort of being in the presence of others might be replaced by a greater comfort with absence, especially with those we don't know intimately. Instead of asking, "Is there a reason to do this online?" we'll be asking, "Is there any good reason to do this in person?" Katherine Mangu-Ward editor-in-chief of *Reason* concurred: "COVID-19 will sweep away many of the artificial barriers to moving more of our lives online... But in many areas of our lives, uptake on genuinely useful online tools has been slowed by powerful legacy players, often working in collaboration with overcautious bureaucrats."

The language necessary to describe this development has yet to mature but it has been referred to as tele-, telework, teleducation, et al. Of course this does not refer to strictly telephone mediated communication any more than the pocket-portable smartphone is really a 'phone'. Rather, any and all electronically mediated communication or, conversely, any non-face-to-face communication (excluding physical mail) might be termed tele- (a misnomer in the spirit of the Black Death and the Spanish flu).

From the point at which the various lockdowns and closures were put in place, countless jobs were moved from the office or the studio to the home. Many will stay there because there are sound long term economic reasons to keep them there that offer benefits to both employers and employees. For an employee, time spent commuting is unpaid labour: a one-hour commute adds two hours to the work day. Working from home also offers the potential for more flexible childcare, better work/life balance and a host of other 'soft' benefits. Employees who rely on public transit may prefer working at home to crowding onto subways and buses. For some individuals telework will not work; they need the discipline of office hours or miss socialising around the water cooler, but for many it will prove ideal.

A spinoff of this trend will be a new demand for home offices. Everyone from contractors and building supply stores to office furniture manufacturers will see secondary benefits from this burgeoning niche in the economy. Similarly, video conferencing apps have seen an explosion in usage. Another beneficial side effect of the trend toward working from home is improvements in air quality. Simply put, fewer commuters means less smog. With growing evidence linking COVID-19 to air quality and generalised concern around global warming, this is one of the more positive consequences of the pandemic.

The true driver for the telework trend will not be employee satisfaction though – it will be the massive savings it provides for corporations. Office space in Manhattan cost an average of 160.90 USD per square foot annually in 2019. Moving 10,000 square feet out of Manhattan and into home offices represents an immediate savings of $1.6 million. And, that is just chump change. Morgan Stanley leases 1.3 million square feet in Manhattan. If it were to reduce that by 10% the savings would amount to 21 million USD annually. The move to Zoom, remote work and home offices is here to stay.

The downside to this development is the class bias implicit in the shift to telework. Most jobs conducive to telework are 'white collar'. A computer programmer can work from home, a construction labourer cannot. A BBC radio host can work from home, a slaughterhouse employee cannot. Acknowledging this class bias, the shift to telework, will be significant for those in eligible professions.

Online shopping ('Teleretail') is booming. Amazon and its ilk cannot hire fast enough but bricks and mortar retailers are falling. Flagship high-end department store Neiman Marcus, based in Dallas, Texas, filed for bankruptcy protection on May 8. In August Lord & Taylor revealed plans to liquidate its stores as soon as they reopened to avoid bankruptcy. Canada has seen a string of similar bankruptcies, epitomised by the demise of iconic shoe retailer Aldo's. In the UK, major high street names such as Debenhams, John Lewis, Burger King and Boots indicated plans to close selected stores nationwide to protect those that remained open. The Centre for Retail Research reported 40 retail bankruptcies in the first six months of 2020, the same number there were in the entire year in 2019. The list includes Oliver Sweeney Trading, the retail subsidiary of the prestige shoe company; Muji, the Japanese homewares retailer; Cardinal, the Yorkshire-based firm of shopfitters; and Soletrader, a footwear retailer.

As the High Street collapses, online shopping is surging. Grocery shopping has traditionally been an online laggard, with consumers worried about freshness. However, the director of Dalhousie University's Agri-food Analytics Lab, Dr Sylvain Charlebois, said the number of Canadians buying food online regularly has quadrupled since the start of the COVID-19 pandemic. In England, online grocer Ocado chief executive Tim Steiner told the BBC, "As a result of COVID-19, we have seen years of growth in the online grocery market condensed into a matter of months; and we won't be going back. We are confident that accelerated growth in the online channel will continue, leading to a permanent redrawing of the landscape of the grocery industry worldwide."

In the wider online marketplace exponential increases were occurring. Amazon launched a campaign to recruit thousands of staff – 3000 in South Africa, 3000 in North Carolina, 2000 at multiple sites across Canada, 2000 in Spain. The growth in online sales has had spinoffs, notably in the courier/delivery business. In Canada, Purolator is adding 1000 employees to meet the demand. Canada Post set a one-day record on May 19, delivering 2.1 million parcels to Canadians, three times the norm for this time of year. The COVID-19 crisis compressed what could have been several years' worth of shifts to online retailers like Amazon and Shopify into a period of weeks.

In a similar fashion, the pandemic did not initiate online education but it has, of necessity, accelerated the process. In the USA the federal government was pressing schools to open in-person classes but encountered strong pushback from the states and local school boards. Canadian provinces encountered resistance from teachers' unions and some parents with a goal of a partial reopening of schools in September but few practical measures were in place. In the UK, there was a brief and limited reopening of schools in early June although some boards refused to do so and dozens of outbreaks were promptly reported thereafter. A full reopening was initiated only at the end of the summer holiday and even then many remained concerned about the safety of both teachers and pupils. For all of these reasons online learning is likely to experience continued growth in the future.

However, this means that economically disadvantaged students are in a hole before classes even start. Online learning carries with it certain assumptions that students without financial means often cannot meet. Online learning requires, at least, a computer; a fast, reliable Internet connection; and, a quiet place to read, study and Zoom or attend online classes. Economically less well-off students can rarely fulfill these unspoken requirements. Canadian journalist Malcolm Gladwell noted that, "virtually all of the advantage that wealthy students have over poor students is the result of differences in the way privileged students learn when they are not in school". With schools closed, economically disadvantaged students, unable to access food programmes, may actually be malnourished also.

Beyond the class barriers presented by online learning, there are a mixed bag of consequences to the shift. An opportunity will be presented by the reduced need for classroom space and school buildings. Could they be converted to community centres or daycare centres? Sold to capitalize the shift to online learning? The possibilities are endless and it is inevitable that a shift to online learning will result in excess physical plant. On the downside, online learning eliminates the social, and socialising experience that is so much a part of education. Whether it is life in residence, athletics, clubs or debate in class, much of this aspect of schooling will be lost. The isolation and lack of the socialisation experience may be particularly damaging to young children. Regardless, schools, particularly universities and colleges, will be compelled to move to online learning.

There is also an indirect economic cost to not opening schools to in class instruction. It is more difficult for parents to return to the workforce if they have children at home. In other words, the push to reopen schools may have more to do with the economy than education or public health. The economy needs children in school so their parents are able to return to work. This may not be the best way to confront a pandemic from a public health point of view, but there are stakeholders who do not see COVID-19 as primarily a public health issue. The downside to this view is that prioritising the economy and reopening too soon can lead to increased transmission and outbreaks. This is a common dilemma during pandemics. Defoe worried about the economic effects of the plague and a century ago ill-advised public gatherings fostered the deadly second wave of influenza. The same debate plays out today as public health officials press for restrictions and counsel an abundance of caution – while others emphasize the need to mitigate the economic impacts.

Telemedicine is one of the moves to electronically mediated communication that will rely on the smartphone. The changes in medical practice will be profound, but the most immediate and the most evident has been the use of the telephone appointment – accompanied by online forms and the ability to instantly send photographs of the patient's afflicted body part where necessary or alternatively an examination by video call.

"The pandemic will shift the paradigm of where our healthcare delivery takes place. For years, telemedicine has lingered on the sidelines as a cost-controlling, high convenience system. Out of necessity, remote office visits could skyrocket in popularity", according to Ezekiel J. Emanuel, chair of the department of medical ethics and health policy at the University of Pennsylvania. There are a host of reasons for this and, again, there are both push and pull factors encouraging this development. For the patient the advantages are self evident. Time off work, travel arrangements; all can be avoided with a tele-appointment. Most importantly, during an infectious respiratory pandemic it eliminates the need to sit in the waiting room. Emanuel added, "There would also be containment-related benefits to this shift; staying home for a video call keeps you out of the transit system, out of the waiting room and, most importantly, away from patients who need critical care." The medical tele-appointment epitomises social distancing.

Government and economy

Working from home and telephone medical appointments are not likely to become contentious issues but the same cannot be said about the move away from face-to-face voting and face-to-face legislating. Like 1918, 2020 is an election year – a presidential election in the United States. At the time of writing it was a campaign fraught with extreme emotions and sentiments, with political opponents framed as enemies and the election sure to be contentious. Voting methods were becoming a key issue and the tolerance and compromise that typified the 1918 ballot was largely absent.

The pandemic will demand changes in polling, namely an increase in means of casting a ballot other than face-to-face at a traditional polling station. Joe Brotherton, of Democracy Live, an online voting startup, told Politico, "One victim of COVID-19 will be the old model of limiting voting to polling places where people must gather in close proximity for an extended period of time." President Trump has argued that voting by mail, the most common form of absentee voting, will result in massive voter fraud, possibly so much so that the result of the election may be invalid.

This position presents voting by mail as a radical or even dangerous departure – yet members of the US military have voted by mail since the Civil War. Many states already permit 'no excuse' absentee voting and the president himself has already voted by mail for the fall election – he recently took up Florida citizenship and cast his vote 'in' Florida.

Brotherton again: "Over the long term, as election officials grapple with how to allow for safe voting in the midst of a pandemic, the adoption of more advanced technology – including secure, transparent, cost-effective voting from our mobile devices – is more likely. In the near-term, a hybrid model – mobile-phone voting with paper ballots for tabulation – is emerging in the 2020 election cycle in certain jurisdictions." Despite the President's claims of fraud, Politico outlined the situation heading into November's election: "In November, 42 states and the District of Columbia will effectively allow for, at a minimum, no-excuse absentee balloting — meaning any voter, regardless of age, health or location on Election Day will be able to vote by mail should they choose to do so. Of those 42 states, just seven are planning to proactively mail every voter a ballot. Five do it as regular course — Colorado, Hawaii, Oregon, Utah and Washington — while California and Vermont, along with Washington D.C., have announced their intention to do so due to the pandemic." Further, according to the US Election Assistance Commission, in 2016 over 57 million Americans cast absentee ballots, meaning 40% of all ballots were cast other than at a polling station. Absentee voting – by mail or mobile phone – is no new procedure and historically has not led to a great deal of voter fraud.

Ultimately, voting will move online. During the pandemic it will move toward absentee ballots, namely mail-in ballots, to avoid the crowding and queues at polling stations. Brotherton concluded, "This system is not an idea; it is a reality that has been used in more than 1000 elections for nearly a decade by our overseas military and disabled voters. This should be the new normal. The shift from paper ballots and polling stations to absentee voting will accelerate in the wake of the pandemic."

The idea of online legislating is considerably more radical. MIT media professor Ethan Zuckerman argues that it offers important benefits beyond the medical. In epidemiological terms social distancing in Congress or Houses of Parliament is impossible with the members seated in tight rows of desks, crowding into committee rooms and confronting media scrums. Already, amid the pandemic, legislatures have moved towards online or hybrid sessions with only a limited number of members present in person. Canada and Britain have some members present in the legislature and others participating virtually. In the US, the House of Representatives has introduced proxy voting but the Senate has refused to do so.

According to Zuckerman, "this is a great time for congresspeople to return to their districts and start the process of virtual legislating – permanently." He argues that there are three specific nonmedical benefits to this change; elected representatives based in their electoral district rather than a distant capital will be more sensitive to local needs; and dispersed in this manner they will be harder to lobby, "as the endless parties and receptions that lobbyists throw in Washington will be harder to replicate across the whole nation". Finally, partisanship and party loyalty could be weakened by dispersal, encouraging members to prioritize local issues over party allegiance. Zuckerman makes a sound argument for tele-legislating, but the proposal is so radical and the pushback will be so strong from vested interests, that it is unlikely to become a permanent change.

A development related to the move online will be the increasing automation of manufacturing and industry. Simply put, machines do not get sick. Any worker whose labour can be automated will find himself replaced. In many factories social distancing is impossible, further incentive to automate. And it's not only factories that will be affected. Grocery stores and supermarkets will increasingly shift to self-checkouts while ATMs will continue to replace bank tellers. Increasingly, any labour that can be automated will be, with machines replacing humans. This is no new development but it will be accelerated by the current pandemic.

A recent economic trend that will be stopped dead in its tracks is the globalisation of supply chains. Seeking ever lower wages and increased efficiencies, corporations have developed ever more complex transnational supply chains. The pandemic has revealed two significant weaknesses with this system. Todd N. Tucker, director of Governance Studies at the Roosevelt Institute, argued that in the circumstances, international supply chains were becoming a threat to national security, "one can imagine a perfect storm in which deep recessions plus mounting geopolitical tensions limit America's access to its normal supply chains and the lack of homegrown capacity in various product markets limits the government's ability to respond nimbly to threats."

In the 2020 crisis the demand for PPE, ventilators and medication revealed that national interests could and would disrupt international supply chains in essential goods. As vaccines are developed the same national interests are going to influence their distribution. Tucker considered that governments would have to become involved more directly in supply chains. "Government has a much bigger role to play in creating adequate redundancy in supply chains – resilient even to trade shocks from allies. This will be a substantial reorientation from even the very recent past," he concluded. On the downside, economist Dambisa Moyo noted, "Switching to a more robust domestic supply chain would reduce dependence on an increasingly fractured global supply system. But while this would better ensure that people get the goods they need, this shift would likely also increase costs." The shift away from transnational supply chains will hit hard-pressed consumers in the pocket.

This issue of a government role in national supply chains raises a larger question of government involvement in wider issues. In broad strokes the past 50 years have seen a move away from Keynesian economics and 'big government' toward neo-liberal, free market economics. Yet the pandemic has revealed the positive role government can play. The crisis has brought public health to the forefront, demanding massive government involvement and investment in vaccine research. Historian Margaret O'Mara has argued that big government will regain its cachet: "The battle against the coronavirus already has made government – federal, state and local – far more visible to Americans... We are seeing the critical role that "big government" plays in our lives and our health." NYT columnist Michiko Kakutani argues that the expertise and professionalism of bureaucrats, denigrated along with big government, will also make a comeback, "A recognition that government institutions – including those entrusted with protecting our health, preserving our liberties and overseeing our national security – need to be staffed with experts (not political loyalists), that decisions need to be made through a reasoned policy process and predicated on evidence-based science and historical and geopolitical knowledge. Institutions, expertise and bureaucracy – personified by doctors Andrew Fauci and Deborah Birx in the USA will regain a respect that has been fading since the 1980s.

Transport and housing

The pandemic will have a revolutionary impact on urban design and cities. Many commuters, working from home permanently, will not return to the urban environment. More importantly, many cities are moving to make their core areas physically more cyclist and pedestrian friendly. Oakland, California has closed 75 miles of its street network to encourage walking and cycling. Chicago, Los Angeles and a host of other American cities have followed suit, as have Berlin, Budapest and Mexico City.

However, it is Milan's Strade Aperte (Open Roads) programme that epitomises the new themes in urban design. Speed limits on most streets have been lowered to 20mph. Twenty-two miles of roadway has been reduced in width to expand cycling and walking opportunities. According to urban planner and former transportation commissioner for New York City, Janette Sadik-Khan, "The Milan plan is so important because it lays out a good playbook for how you can reset your cities now. It's a once-in-a-lifetime opportunity to take a fresh look at your streets and make sure that they are set to achieve the outcomes that we want to achieve: not just moving cars as fast as possible from point A to point B, but making it possible for everyone to get around safely." In Milan and many other cities the changes are planned to remain when the pandemic abates. In this sense the outbreak has fundamentally and radically altered cities – permanently undermining car culture.

In the same way that walking and cycling have become higher priorities in a post-COVID-19 world, so too urban green space will grow in importance. Alexandra Lange, architecture critic at Curbed, has pointed out that the National Trust in Britain is increasing access during the lockdown and noted that daily walks through Brooklyn Bridge Park and along the Brooklyn Heights Promenade have been key to her wellbeing during the lockdown. Cholera directly led to Baron Haussmann's redesign of Paris and influenced Frederick Law Olmsted's views on parks as the lungs of the city. This pandemic will result in cities more oriented towards pedestrians, bicycle lanes and urban greenspace.

On the downside of this move away from the automobile is the anomalous position of public transit. Social distancing is impossible on a crowded subway in Manhattan or a bus in London. Additionally, there is the problem of frequently touched railings, handholds, ticket machines, etc. This perceived risk will discourage public transit use. According to Ahsan Habib, director of the school of planning at Dalhousie University, massive investment will be required to make public transit safe in the wake of COVID-19: "We need new terminals, we need new markings, new seating arrangements." Going forward, viable public transit will require new policies and procedures, and investment in infrastructure – otherwise many potential riders will perceive it to be too risky.

This pandemic will send major aftershocks through urban real estate markets. There will be a significant decrease in demand both commercially and residentially. If 30% fewer workers are coming to the office because they have chosen to work from home there will be a corresponding drop in demand for office space. In June, Politico Brief opined that with the drop in demand, "there will probably be a crash in real estate values in the coming weeks and months". Calgary-based real estate professional John Brown reported already seeing that effect in the market, "I'm having a number of conversations with companies that are saying, 'We may not need the space that we have.'" A recession coupled with an increase in working from home will have a significant negative impact on urban commercial real estate.

The pandemic will have a similar negative impact on the urban residential real estate market, specifically condominiums and strata living. Two specific aftereffects of the pandemic will drive down prices. First, with the increase in telework, fewer employees will need to live in urban areas. In the English real estate market, sales listings in London are increasing while demand for homes outside the city is growing. Like the royal court in 1665, in an age of zoonotic viruses many who can afford to are leaving the city. Also, many condominiums in markets such as Toronto and London are owned by investors who never planned on living in their units but rather, always intended to let them as short-term rentals and have Airbnb guests pay the mortgage. Tourist travel and business travel will shrink after the pandemic and these investments may not play out the way their owners had planned. Many condominium investors will find themselves forced to sell at the same time as demand declines. This foretells a significant drop in prices.

That said, the private housing market in the UK remained buoyant as households tired of looking at the interior of their home for months at a time during lockdown looked to change their scenery.

Travel and tourism

One of the most conspicuous casualties of the lockdown has been the aviation industry. The previously thriving business of air travel collapsed as governments impose travel bans and quarantines, forcing airlines to mothball their expensive aircraft. When journeys resumed, airlines were initially leaving the middle seat empty but even that concession ended for financial reasons. Rather, passengers were required to wear masks and face shields. Eventually there were plans for significant changes ranging from walk-through sanitizers before boarding to barriers between seats. To save money and eliminate 'touchpoints' (contact between staff and passengers) inflight service was being curtailed. Singapore Airlines, long renowned for its service, has eliminated inflight meals and substituted a bagged lunch on boarding to reduce staff/passenger contact. As is the case with public transit, the communal nature of flying will increase the perception of risk, and discourage recreational travellers. Many business trips, as noted earlier, will become Zoom calls – further depressing passenger numbers. The future is not bright for the airline industry.

The ripple effects of this on tourist destinations will roll across the globe from Malta and Ibiza to Alaska and the Caribbean. In these destinations, hotels and short term rentals will sit empty because guests are unwilling to fly there. Fly-in fishing and hunting camps, significant industries in the North American wilderness, face this insurmountable problem coupled with community resistance to 'outsiders' possibly bringing in the disease. The first case in Haida Gwai, an isolated aboriginal territory off the north shore of British Columbia, ignited finger pointing and accusations. Along the coast indigenous communities have imposed travel and tourism bans to protect their communities.

In a fascinating response, Barbados is encouraging Canadians working from home to make their 'home' in Barbados. The Barbados Welcome

Stamp grants a one-year work visa to Canadians for a fee of 3000 CAD. Interestingly, the lead on this initiative is not an economic ministry but rather Barbados Tourism Marketing Inc. (BTMI). The hope is that takers will need accommodation, dine in restaurants and partially fill the tourist void. Taking advantage of the programme, like many COVID-19 consequences, has distinct socioeconomic limits. The programme is, inevitably, restricted to people able to work from home and requires a 2019 income tax return proving an income of at least 50,000 CAD.

Cruise lines also face a bleak future. American late-night host Stephen Colbert referred to them as 'floating petri dishes' and their experience during the beginning of the 2020 pandemic was not encouraging. On multiple occasions, COVID-19 raced through the passengers and crew while the ships sat isolated in ports or offshore in locations around the world. This can hardly be regarded as surprising – consider the footprint of a cruise ship and the number of guests and crew, crammed into it. On land, such density would be considered a tenement. The close quarters nature of a cruise ship coupled with their disastrous experiences during this pandemic will deal a heavy blow to the industry.

Cruise ships also bring up the issue of shared air. As SARS and the Metropole Hotel in Hong Kong demonstrated, 'shared air' can be infectious. Merely being on the same floor of a hotel was enough to infect 17 people. Similarly, an investigation conducted in a restaurant in China during the current pandemic demonstrated that air currents in the dining area (created by an air conditioning unit) influenced which patrons were and were not infected. On a cruise ship, with most cabins having no windows, recycled air is unavoidable and, potentially, dangerous.

The implications of this issue are profound. It could impact on heating, ventilation and air conditioning (HVAC) systems in myriad fields. Will it be safe to stroll through, and shop in, an indoor mall? How safe is strata living if the building is heated by hot air? Most buildings create positive air pressure in units and exhaust into the hallways and common areas. So how safe will the hallways be if even a single resident is infected? At the Metropole none of the infected had any contact with the original superspreader; they only used the same hallways. And what does that imply for the safety of hotels going forward?. What does this mean for office towers where thousands of workers from dozens of different companies share air? In June the Journal of the American Medical Association published an article by two Harvard Medical School doctors arguing that air flow and air disinfection were misunderstood and underestimated as to their role in transmission. This is almost a grey elephant: its implications are so profound there is a temptation to refuse to even consider it.

The industry is already working towards solutions however. Increased filtration has been proposed but its effectiveness is questionable and it would require larger blowers to force the air through any filters installed. Alternately, bands of UV light have been proposed to kill the virus. The only other alternative if air disinfection is a serious issue would be to move to hot water or radiant electric heat and totally eliminate HVAC systems and 'shared air'. Regardless, any modifications would be extraordinarily expensive.

Sports and leisure

Social distancing has also proven to be extremely difficult for the hospitality and entertainment industries. All businesses in these fields rely on numbers for their profits and often margins are thin. Theatres often require 70% occupancy to make a profit. Filling only one-third of the seats will make the business model unsustainable.

Restaurants face the same issues. It is a notoriously difficult industry, known for its razor thin margins and frequent failures. In Chicago, the famous Michelin-starred Blackbird has closed permanently. The *New Orleans Picayune Times* reported, "The Louisiana Restaurant Association projects one in four restaurants statewide could close permanently. For the New Orleans area that forecast is much worse, rising to 40% to 50% closing, due to the city's heavy reliance on travel and events." Paul Prudhomme's K-Paul's Louisiana Kitchen, a fixture in the heart of the French Quarter of New Orleans since 1979, announced its permanent closure in early July. The temporary shutdowns and ongoing social distancing will hit every segment of the restaurant industry.

American cultural critic Alex Rawls expressed concern about the impact of the pandemic on live music. He saw 'drive-in' concerts and other stop gaps being experimented with as unsustainable and worried that reduced seating to maintain social distancing would force live venues to raise ticket prices so high that attending a concert would become a 'prestige event', akin to attending the World Cup or the Superbowl: affordable only for the super rich.

Professional sports faces an uncertain future to say the least. Sporting bodies are under intense pressure to reopen for multiple reasons – not least because they are at the centre of vast industries with revenues derived not only from ticket sales but also from television rights, advertising and merchandising. This income supports not only the teams and their owners but also the broadcast networks and advertisers, athletes and stadium personnel, security and police officers. In North America, President Trump wanted them up and operating as the presidential election drew near. Interviewed on July 22, 2020, Dr Alan Davidson, an infectious disease researcher at the U of Toronto and a Baltimore Orioles fan, was not optimistic about major league baseball's then-recent restart. He predicted that "they'll play a few games and have to shut it down because of an outbreak." Within a week an Orioles series against the Florida Marlins had to be cancelled because of an outbreak on that team which saw 17 infected. There is a risk to players on the field in every sport, but the greatest risk will be in the dressing rooms and clubhouses as evidenced by the Marlins outbreak.

The NHL has restarted in 'bubbles' in two Canadian cities, the NFL has opened training camps and some soccer leagues have resumed play with one big 'but': they are playing in empty stadiums. For most leagues ticket revenue is minor compared to broadcast revenue and this is of little concern. However, Canadian Football League (CFL) clubs rely primarily on ticket revenue and this situation looked set to devastate them. In the longer term, teams risk losing fan interest if the live experience vanishes and professional sports become a purely televisual experience. In the here and now, like major league baseball, attempts to restart professional sports are doomed to failure.

The FIA and Formula 1 continued to race in 2020, testing all personnel connected with the motorsport on a regular basis. Between July 17 and July 23, 1461 drivers, mechanics, team members and associated personnel were tested for COVID-19 and there were no positive results. However, Racing Point driver Sergio Perez was ruled out of the British Grand Prix after testing positive following a visit to his mother in Mexico.

In football, there were reportedly several cases of COVID-19 in English Premier League players during the summer break and from September the league was set to begin publishing the results of regular testing.

Global effects

All of the discussion of sequelae to this point has focused on immediate, direct and specific impacts. However, there are two looming issues that are of greater import than all of these issues combined. The overall economic impact of this pandemic will be as significant as that of the Black Death, although the ways in which this will manifest are entirely different. Internationally, the pandemic's effect on the difficult and deteriorating US-China relationship will be profound.

Economically, the Black Death shifted the balance of power between labourers and landlords in favour of the former and wages rose. There is no reason to believe that will happen this time. Currently unemployment figures are astronomical. The Pew Research Center put it simply, "Unemployment rose higher in three months of COVID-19 than it did in two years of the Great Recession." An accompanying report noted the truth was worse because, "Unemployment rate is higher than officially recorded, more so for women and certain other groups." In the UK the BBC reported in mid-July, "The number of employees paying tax fell by 649,000 from March to June. Average earnings fell, and the average number of hours people worked dropped by a record amount, according to figures for March to May." This pandemic will not drive wages up.

McKinsey & Company, the American management consulting firm has produced nine macroeconomic scenarios for a post-COVID world. In a best case scenario including successful non-pharmaceutical virus suppression and prompt discovery and production of a vaccine they estimate that annual global GDP will decline between four and five trillion USD. Their worst case scenario sees a 20 trillion USD decline. A massive economic contraction is unavoidable. Consequently, there will be an excess of labour. From waiters to airline pilots, unemployment will be widespread, the diametric opposite of the aftermath of the Black Death. Corporate bankruptcies will also soar. NYU finance professor and bankruptcy expert Walter I Altman told the NYT that mega bankruptcies — filings by companies with $1 billion or more in debt will set a record in 2020 at 66 and large bankruptcies — at least $100 million — may surpass the previous high set in the aftermath of the 2008 economic crisis.

Attempts to address the increase in unemployment, bankruptcies and declining GDP governments have been forced to offer huge relief packages to address everything from individual unemployment to iconic industry players such as Boeing, suddenly and unexpectedly facing insolvency. This has led to expensive legislation that suddenly has everyone across the political spectrum in favour of government deficits. Consequently, McKinsey & Co estimate that, globally, government deficits could reach 30 trillion USD by 2023. The devil is always in the details and beyond issues of the fairness of the various programmes in their distribution the ultimate question will be who pays the bill. In the broadest sense there are two paths. Governments can preach austerity or they can seriously, structurally alter their financing, rather than their finances.

The former road would emphasise cutting social services and unemployment programmes (at a time of soaring unemployment) to reduce government expenditures. The alternative would involve increasing government revenue through estate or death taxes, higher corporate tax rates and taxing the 'super rich'. In the midst of the pandemic this latter option, the road less travelled, has garnered support from an unlikely, but influential, group: the super-rich themselves. In mid-July 2020, 83 of the world's richest people wrote a letter arguing they should be taxed more.

They acknowledged that they were hardly frontline workers, "No, we are not the ones caring for the sick in intensive care wards. We are not driving the ambulances that will bring the ill to hospitals. We are not restocking grocery store shelves or delivering food door to door". They then noted that this did not prevent them from playing a role, "But we do have money, lots of it. Money that is desperately needed now and will continue to be needed in the years ahead, as our world recovers from this crisis."

In the UK, the Labour party has proposed a wealth tax on the super rich to fund the recovery from COVID-19. Defoe and Boccacio remarked on a meaner, more self-indulgent world in the wake of their pandemics. If that proves true in the present case the idea of an outcome that seriously addresses the growing wealth gap and reverses that trend might seem unlikely. On the other hand, perhaps, this represents a paradigm shift in views of the governmental role and government financing. It is certainly the first time a serious candidate for the Democrat presidential nomination has argued for a basic income (Andrew Wang).

Ultimately, it may depend on perception, in the sense that all politics is psychology. Optimists will look forward to a changed post-COVID-19 world where income distribution is less extreme and social service rates exceed the poverty line. Pessimists, on the other hand, will be inclined to see a future of austerity in response to soaring government debt. Also, there are bound to be national variations in approach. A Scandinavian country is more likely to adopt a socialist leaning solution than a government in the United States. The only thing clear about the future of the economy is that it will be bleak, characterised by bankruptcies, unemployment, consequent foreclosures and evictions, and soaring government debt for years to come.

The shifting power relationship between China and the US is clearer. It is apparent that the United States is being bested – despite the fact that the disease originated in China and the US administration is making every effort to hang the handle 'Chinese virus' on SARS-CoV-2. This change in the balance of power began long ago and increased when President Trump was elected in 2016. In classic pandemic fashion it has accelerated in the last six months.

In early August 2020, US Health Secretary Alex Azar visited Taiwan to discuss COVID-19 and medical supplies with his Taiwanese counterparts. He is the highest level American official to visit Taiwan since 1979 and the visit has more to do with challenging China than public health. Similarly, the White House continues to bandy about the term 'Chinese virus' with no objective other than to offend the Chinese. According to Pew they are succeeding – with a majority of Americans blaming China for the virus, and almost 80% convinced they are responsible for the virus's spread. That said, Trump's personal approval rating has plummeted as the COVID-19 death toll has climbed in the USA.

Most importantly, while picking pointless fights with China, Trump has also withdrawn the USA from the world stage as China has increased its influence. Symbolic of this, and directly related to the pandemic, was the US withdrawal of support for the WHO. The US complained that the WHO did not pressure China to respond more forcefully and be more open in the early stages of the pandemic.

This may be true, but the WHO has no enforcement powers, relying on cooperation and persuasion alone. Regardless, in April Trump announced that the US was suspending WHO funding; in May he announced that the US was withdrawing from the organisation; and, in July, the US announced its formal withdrawal effective July 2021. This policy effectively cedes the field to China. Absent the US, China's influence in the organisation can only increase. Every time Trump has disparaged allies, denigrated NATO and further isolated the United States, he has given ground to China. The incoherent and ineffective response to the pandemic has further undermined America's international profile. Additionally, Trump's 'America first' mantra may taint America's image when vaccines are discovered and distributed. Already the EU, the UK and the USA have preordered millions of doses of potential vaccines for their own citizens, leaving poor countries at the back of the bus. In this kind of competitive environment it would be foolish to believe Trump would perform honourably or cooperatively.

Whether Trump will still be president if and when a vaccine reaches the point of mass production is unclear at the time of writing. Yet whoever is resident in the White House, while the 20th century could be characterised as the 'American century', it appears increasingly likely that the 21st century will be the 'Chinese century'. The pandemic has simply hastened this change.

As an undergraduate at the University of Toronto, the author had the opportunity to meet a man called Jan Karski. In 1942, as a soldier in the Polish Home Army, he was twice smuggled by tunnel into the Warsaw ghetto to report on conditions. Wearing the uniform of a bribed Estonian auxiliary he also worked a shift inside a sorting camp for the Bełżec and Sobibor death camps. He was subsequently spirited out of occupied Europe to inform the world. His eyewitness testimony was taken seriously, seriously enough to earn him an audience with President Roosevelt. When Karski finished his presentation, Roosevelt brushed him off on Supreme Court Justice Felix Frankfurter. Only recently appointed to the Supreme Court, Frankfurter had spent years as a close and trusted adviser of the president. He was a man who could deliver a message, unofficially and indirectly, that came straight from the White House. In the Polish embassy, he told Karski, "I cannot believe you." Frankfurter was informing Karski that the veracity of his tale was not in doubt, but there was no response possible and, therefore, the problem, the genocidal reality of the Holocaust, would not be acknowledged.

The situation is painfully analogous to the state of pandemic planning in the pre-COVID-19 world. As soon as the nature of the virus and the rapidity of its spread became apparent there were immediate, flashing red lights within government bureaucracies. Warnings explicitly stated that it was a question of when, not if. Academics, from microbiologists to historians and geographers, had been warning that a pandemic would overwhelm the healthcare system, savage the economy and discombobulate society for decades. There were even close calls and dry runs from, SARS and MERS to Ebola and H1N1; an alphabet soup of almosts. Unfortunately, viewing the odds through an electoral lens, politicians repeatedly bet that the pandemic of the century would not happen on their watch. They were warned, felt for their pocketbooks, and said, 'We cannot believe you.' We are now paying the price for their decisions and the values underlying those decisions.

Going forward, it is essential to understand that saying, 'I cannot believe you' is no longer an option. Even if we were to discover a perfect vaccine and eradicate SARS-CoV-2 it would not be the end. Zoonosis is here to stay and it will happen again and again, with increasing frequency. Winston Churchill's quote from another war and another century is apropos: "Now this is not the end. It is not even the beginning of the end. But it is, perhaps, the end of the beginning."

> *"'It was plague. We've had the plague here.'*
> *You'd almost think they expected to be given medals for it.*
> *But what does that mean, 'plague'?*
> *Just life, no more than that."*
>
> The Plague, Albert Camus

Glossary

Aedes (Ae. aegypti and Ae. albopictus) – Species of mosquitoes; vectors for zika, dengue and yellow fever.

Asymptomatic – The time (hours, days, or weeks) between when a person is first exposed to an infection or virus and when the first symptoms (like coughing or fever) begin. During this period an individual may unknowingly infect others.

Black Death – see Plague.

Case Fatality Rate (CFR) – The proportion of individuals who die from a pandemic virus as a function of only those infected (total number of people who die of the virus divided by total number of people who are infected; multiply by 100 to get percentage). Also known as mortality rate.

Cholera – An acute secretory diarrhea caused by infection with the bacterium Vibrio cholerae.

Clinical Attack Rate (CAR) – Percentage of population that gets sick from a virus (e.g. 20,000 cases of influenza in a population of 100,000 people equals a 20% CAR). Also, known as morbidity rate.

Community mitigation strategy – A strategy designed to slow down or limit the transmission of a pandemic virus in a community.

Contact transmission – The spread of an infectious agent caused by physical contact of a susceptible host with people or objects.

Cordon sanitaire – A guarded line preventing anyone from leaving an area infected by a disease and thus spreading it.

Coronavirus – a family of virus that includes SARS-CoV, MERS-CoV and SARS-CoV-2.

COVID-19 – The disease caused by the SARS-CoV-2 virus.

Droplet transmission – The spread of an infectious agent caused by the dissemination of droplets. Droplets are generated by an infected person during coughing, sneezing and talking. Transmission occurs when these droplets that contain microorganisms are propelled, up to two yards, through the air and deposited on the mucosa of another person.

Dysentery – Shigellosis is an infectious disease caused by a group of bacteria called Shigella (shih-GEHL-uh). Most who are infected with Shigella develop diarrhea, fever, and stomach cramps starting a day or two after they are exposed to the bacteria.

Ebola – A severe and often fatal zoonotic infectious hemorrhagic fever in humans and other mammals emerged in the Congo.

Endemic – A disease that is constantly present at low levels within a community, population or region.

Epidemic – A disease that affects a large number of people within a community, population, or region.

Essential goods – Food and other supplies that are necessary to survive, such as medical supplies and gasoline.

Essential services – Services and functions that must be continued, even during a pandemic, to maintain health and welfare.

Hand hygiene – Frequent handwashing with soap and water for 20 seconds and use of hand sanitiser to reduce contact transmission. Frequent hand-washing or use of alcohol-based products (gels, rinses, foams) that do not require the use of water.

Immunity – The ability to avoid infection or disease through the body's immune system. Immunity can be innate (present at or around birth) or acquired, either through exposure to disease or through vaccination.

Influenza – Influenza (flu) is a contagious respiratory illness caused by influenza viruses. It can cause mild to severe illness. The influenza A and B viruses that routinely spread in people (human influenza viruses) are responsible for seasonal flu epidemics each year.

Intubation – the insertion of an artificial ventilation tube into the trachea tube in order to attach the patient to a ventilator.

Human Immunodeficiency Virus/Acquired Immune Deficiency Syndrome (HIV/AIDS) – a chronic, potentially life-threatening condition caused by the human immunodeficiency virus (HIV) that impairs the human immune system (AIDS).

Mask, Surgical – Disposable face mask that covers the mouth and nose, used to prevent the transmission of germs in medical settings.

Mask, N95 or P2/P3 – An N95 respirator (P2 or P3 in Europe) is a respiratory protective device designed to achieve a very close facial fit and very efficient filtration of airborne particles. The 'N95' designation means that when subjected to careful testing, the respirator blocks at least 95 percent of very small (0.3 micron) test particles. Properly fitted, the filtration capabilities of N95 respirators exceed those of surgical masks. They are essential for processes such as intubation.

Middle East Respiratory Syndrome (MERS-CoV) – Coronavirus that spilled over from dromedary camels. It is highly fatal but only mildly infectious.

Morbidity rate – The number of people in a population who have a disease at a given time (e.g. 20,000 cases of influenza in a population of 100,000 people equals a 20% morbidity rate).

Mortality rate – The number of people in a population who die from a pandemic virus (e.g. 4000 deaths of influenza in a population of 100,000 people equals a 4% mortality rate).

Non-Pharmaceutical Interventions – Non-medical actions that can limit the spread of a disease, such as social distancing and infection control.

Pandemic – An epidemic occurring worldwide or over a wide area, crossing boundaries of several countries, and usually affecting a large number of people.

Plague, Bubonic – A bacterial disease that attacks the lymph system producing black buboes. Fleas carry it from rats to humans and from human to human. The Black Death (1347-1353) was bubonic plague.

Plague, Pneumonic – Bubonic plague that has invaded the respiratory system. Human to human droplet transmission is possible.

Plague, Septicemic – Bubonic plague that has invaded the circulatory system. Human to human droplet transmission is not possible.

Quarantine – Keeping people who may have been exposed to an illness but are not yet sick away from others for a long enough period of time to determine if they are going to get the illness, in order to prevent the spread of the disease.

Reservoir – A host population that provides a pool that keeps the virus population alive. Dromedary camels are a reservoir for MERS-CoV.

Respiratory hygiene – Covering the mouth and nose while coughing or sneezing by using the elbow, shoulder, or disposable tissues to reduce droplet transmission.

R-nought number (Rx) – The number of persons an infected person infects: a key to modelling an epidemic (R3 means one infected person infects 3 others, R1 means one infected person infects one other). The higher the R-nought number, the more rapidly an infectious disease is spreading.

SARS-CoV – The coronavirus that caused the pandemic in 2003.

SARS-CoV-2 – The virus that causes COVID-19.

Self-isolation – Self-imposed isolation by individuals that may have been infected, generally for a period of two weeks.

Sequelae – outcomes, conditions or consequences arising from a disease.

Severe acute respiratory syndrome (SARS) – The first coronavirus pandemic (2003). It spread from Guangdong province, China to Hong Kong and then by air to Singapore, Hanoi and Toronto.

Social distancing – Measures to increase the space (usually a minimum of 7ft or 2m) between people. May include school closures, work closures, and cancellation of public gatherings.

Spanish Flu – A misnomer for the 1918-1919 influenza pandemic.

Typhus – A disease caused by a bacteria called Rickettsia prowazekii. Epidemic typhus is spread to people through contact with infected body lice.

Vaccination – Actually getting the injection or taking an oral vaccine dose. Immunisation refers to becoming immune to the disease following vaccination.

Vector – A species that is an avenue of transmission for an infectious disease. Fleas are a vector for bubonic plague and mosquitoes are a vector for yellow fever.

Vibrio cholerae – The bacteria that causes cholera. It relies on oral-fecal transmission.

Yellow Fever – A viral infection transmitted by mosquitoes. It devastated Napoleon's expeditionary force to Saint-Domingue in 1803.

Yersinia pestis – The flea that is a route of transmission for bubonic plague.

Zoonosis – Disease transmission from animals to the human population. The source of viruses from the 1890 influenza, through HIV to SARS-CoV-2.

Image Credits

1 H. Zell via Wikimedia Commons. Licence: CC BY-SA 3.0
2 Luigi Sabatelli the Elder via Wellcome Collection. Licence: CC BY 4.0
3 Hans Holbein via Wikimedia Commons. Licence: Public domain
4 Hans Holbein via Wikimedia Commons. Licence: Public domain
5 Edward Matthew Ward via Wellcome Collection, ref no. 6425i. Licence: CC BY 4.0
6 Robert Pollard via Wellcome Collection, ref no. 6923i. Licence: CC BY 4.0
7 Paul Fürst via Wikipedia. Licence: Public domain
8 Jules-Élie Delauney via Minneapolis Institute of Art, Gift of Mr. and Mrs. Atherton Bean, Accession no. 72.128. Licence: Public domain
9 Adolph Northen via Wikimedia Commons. Licence: Public domain
10 Charles Minard via Wikipedia. Licence: Public domain
11 Anon via Wellcome Collection. Licence: CC BY 4.0
12 William S. Farr via Centre for Evidence Based Medicine at Oxford University. Licence: Public domain
13 John Leech, Punch magazine via Wikimedia Commons. Licence: Public domain
14 John Snow via Wikimedia Commons. Licence: Public domain
15 Anon via Library and Archives Canada / PA-025025. Licence: Copyright expired
16 Anon, St Louis Post Dispatch via Wikimedia Commons. Licence: Public domain
17 Anon via CDC. Licence: Public domain
18 Phoenix7777 via Wikimedia Commons. Licence: CC BY-SA 4.0
19 John O'Neill via Wikimedia Commons. Licence: CC BY-SA 3.0
20 Alissa Eckert, MSMI; Dan Higgins, MAMS via CDC. Licence: Public domain